Lighten Up

An everyday approach to being healthy, *and* possibly skinny, without obsessing, depriving or pretending to like green juice.

First Published September 2014
By: Colette Maat
             Wellington
             New Zealand

Website: www.coachcolette.com
Linkedin: Linkedin/ColetteMaat
Twitter: @ColetteMaat
Google+:   CoachColetteMaat

Cover and Content Illustrations : Hannah Maat

Dedication

To my dear Mum, whose love of food made her kitchen the ultimate soulful and nourishing place to be. Your memory lives on in my kitchen and will continue to make me smile.

"Stop sitting there with your hands folded looking on, doing nothing; Get into action and live this full and glorious life. Now. You have to do it."
Eileen Caddy
The Dawn of Change

Acknowledgements

Lighten Up has taken me on all sorts of journeys. From journeys of self doubt and procrastination, to hope, excitement, accomplishment and pride.
So my first acknowledgement is to Colette Teresa McNally-Maat. You did what you said you would do and that's great!

To my friend Tina, who planted the seed for this book after sharing one of my lunches, which I'd thrown together with whatever ingredients I had in my pantry at the time.

To My dear friend Sue, whose journalistic eye meant that I had nowhere to hide. For your encouragement, cheerleading and belief in me. And for your willingness to be an inspiration by jumping onboard the 'healthy train'.

To my dear friends and fellow Coaches, Dianne, Cheryl, Cynthia & Ami. You never doubted that I could follow through, especially when I wanted to give up so many times. Your support and guidance is beyond what anyone could wish for.

To Francesca, Michelle and Sue, for giving me a peek into what your food intake in a typical day looks like.

To my dear friend Geoff. Your tips on 'shortening my sentences' made me lose *some* of the drivel and speak on purpose. I hope I have done you proud.

To Anna, Stu and Nigel, for your words of endorsement and for being inspirational in your fields of expertise.

To my loving and patient Husband Aad. Your belief in me never waned. Your patience and support never faltered. I am forever grateful.

Finally and most importantly, to my beautiful, clever and creative daughter *and* illustrator, Hannah. You are my inspiration for living life in health and in love. I love you to infinity. May you inspire many by being your amazing self.

INTRODUCTION

One of my greatest wishes for you whilst creating this book, is that you will be able to easily understand the guidance I have presented throughout. My intention is not to provide you with another 'diet book' or a 'quick fix one week wonder'. In fact, far from it. I want you to enjoy life on your own terms, with a little helping hand along the way. I will not be blinding you with science, or suggesting that you take on a daily Bikram Yoga practice accompanied by litres of green liquid that I would not be prepared to guzzle myself.
I want you to be able to 'flick the switch' without necessarily needing to know how to 'wire the circuit'. I will be addressing some of your physical niggles, busy schedules and budgeting struggles, as well as planting the seed to a healthier legacy for you, for your children and your children's children.

I will also include snippets of my own life, growing up in an Irish Catholic Family on a rural Dairy Farm in Northern Ireland. I share how my environment played such a huge role in my perspective on health, food and on what's really important.

I am a passionate Mum, who cares about the outcome of the choices which make our society sick & tired, obese and, in the extreme, dead! However, I am not a Doctor, Dietitian nor a Psychologist.

If I can help, even just a few of the many, who are heading down the road to ruins in terms of the health choices they make, then I rest easy.

I applaud the efforts of so many who are already waking up by taking responsibility and turning their wellbeing around. By picking up this book, I include you in my applause.

Awareness, or lack there of, isn't necessarily the big issue. My guess is that you know already, or have a pretty good idea, that 'fries & pies' *on a regular basis*, probably isn't the way to go for the health and vitality you adorn to.

So it is a matter of getting used to alternatives and implementing them into your busy life in ways which won't break the bank and without giving up taste. Having said that, I thoroughly believe that you should never 'deprive' yourself of the things you love.

Contradictory as that may sound, statistics have proven that the first thing which will make anyone reach for their favourite item on their craving list, is someone telling them they can't have it. That's human nature!

By starting to take back the steering wheel of your long term health, you no longer have to be answerable to the 'weekly weigh ins', the deprivation that has been recommended by the latest celebrity craze, or the countless dollars spent on exotic supplementation that has been derived from the extract of a rhino's horn! What remains is personal power and informed choices that originate from your intuitive and unique self.

Whilst this book is laid out in 12 sequential chapters, I also invite you to pick it up and jump straight into which ever chapter resonates with you at the time.

CONTENTS:

1. Where do I start?

First of all, you have already made a start. Just by being interested enough to pick up this book, you're further ahead than you think!

The starting point is to clear out your pantry. *You may also refer to your pantry as the larder or food cupboard, depending on where you originate from. As my place of residence at the time of writing this book is New Zealand, I am referring to the 'home of my food' as the 'pantry'.*

Clearing out your pantry

The pantry can be a minefield of confusion when you're busy, hungry and perhaps having the added chaos of kids screaming for their after school infamous 'afternoon tea'.
Mind you, that kind of behaviour will have to be addressed in another book entitled 'Respect for Mum' or 'Teaching Patience to Our Young'!

The first thing I would recommend that you do, is to make 'space'.
It is, I'm afraid, going to be a 'clutter clearing' project. This in itself, is not only one of the most therapeutic and satisfying projects to take on, whether you admit to liking it or not, but one of vital importance when it

comes to a food cupboard. It is a little like clearing out your handbag, only on a much bigger scale!

It would be a good idea to start this project at a time when you can give it your undivided attention. Ideally, this should really only take about an hour or so, depending of course on the size and current state of your pantry. So if you're a busy Mum with school going kids, do it when they're in school. If you have a toddler running around, do it when they are having a nap or when they have their safe play, so you can keep a close eye on them.
If you are a busy executive who spends much less time at home, then the chances are, your pantry will be relatively untouched, therefore needing minimal attention. If this is you, it should be easy to steal 30 minutes on a weekend to tackle this little project. An orderly pantry may well inspire you to host social gatherings around some hearty home cooked creations.

Always begin at the top shelf, working your way down, removing *every* item. Every single little remnant of old christmas puddings which were stashed there in 1999, never to be shown the light of day. Remove the secret stash of your favourite confectionery which has been hidden and out of reach from the beady eyes of little people.
At risk of stating the obvious, please use a safe set of steps or secure footing to reach the high shelves!
Ensure that you can reach into the furthest corners and clean out all the dust, powder and crumbs that you have

been completely unaware of and have really no idea at this stage where they originated from.

So now its empty, everything's on the kitchen work top, resembling the times when you've lost something and in order to find it, you emptied the entire contents of the chest of drawers or equivalent, only to shove it back in with a vow to 'see to it later'.

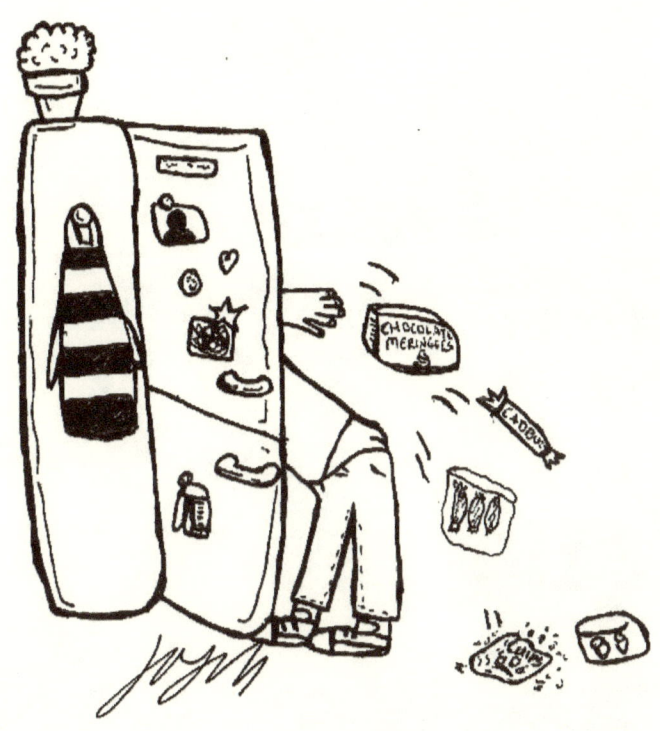

Not Forgetting about the Fridge!

Just when you thought you'd made it into the world of clutter free spaces, your attention now needs to shift to the fridge (refrigerator).

While you are still on a roll, with the momentum of an approaching twister, get to work on doing the exact same process for the contents of the chill box in the corner, using the same guidelines as for your pantry. Where did that cheese appear from anyway? *How long*? You know the drill. Good, that's done!

2. Stocking Up.

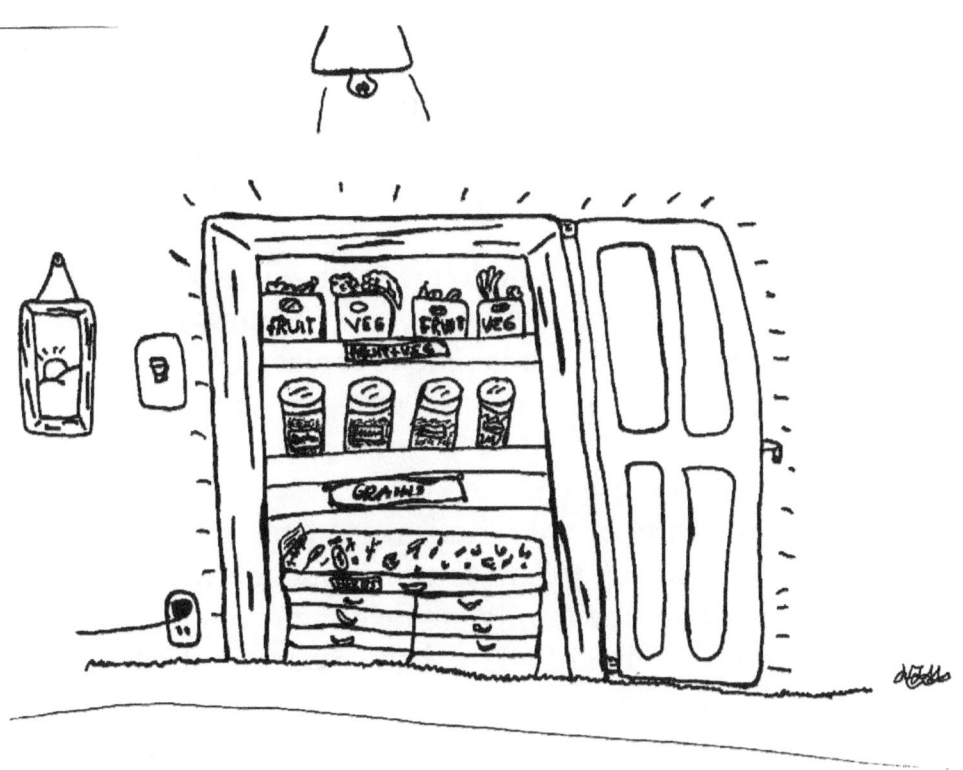

With the pantry and fridge shelves empty and clean, now is the perfect time to do a little date checking. When was the last time you used that box of cornflour? or the tinned peaches? or the jar of pickles?(which should have ideally been stored in the fridge). It's surprising how much you can actually get rid of, guilt free, during this process. By the way, packets of tea and tea bags also have a sell by date!

A word of conscious awareness here. If there is anything which is out of date and is packaged in either plastic, glass or tin, do the right thing and bin the contents, wash the container out and recycle. That little bit of awareness can bring a whole lot of satisfaction to what would otherwise be a nagging thought such as "perhaps I should have......". Now it's done and your conscience is squeaky clean, so let's move forward.

Once you've ditched the no longer edible items, items which have passed their sell by date, or items which you may never actually use, it is time to replace the stock which is in date and is very soon going to be in perfect order.

I would suggest putting some kind of practical approach to the organisation of your foodstuffs. One that not only suits your day to day practical needs, but one where other members of the family are taken into consideration. Think of all the items you would rather see little fingers stay away from. To avoid frustrating moments of negotiation, allocate these items to the top shelf where they remain out of sight.

I have personally tried this with my own daughter, which is why I know it works so well. I noticed that whatever did manage to catch her eye, it immediately became firmly registered in focus and resulted in several negotiating tactics. By keeping the offending culprits out of sight, it creates a lot more harmony and less chance of unnecessary upset. The same applies to all those 'nutritionally questionable' items which have a habit of appearing in the 'goodie bag' brought home from the infamous birthday parties.

My approach in dealing with these situations, was to allow one or two small items from the gift bag, at most. The remaining and often multicoloured stash, would be stored in jar which would become a 'sweet jar/box'. The jar/box would then placed on the highest shelf possible and taken down only on occasions when chores were completed to an outstanding level (I have very high expectations and run a tight ship!), or on an occasion which would be decided by either parent.

What I noticed by doing this, is that they are very often forgotten about and on the occasions when treats are on the agenda, an alternative healthier option can be given.

Since we have now converted your pantry into a form of a sacred space, let's re-stock with some basic and fundamental goodies.

Stocking up on essentials
Although it sounds simplistic and somewhat routine, stocking up requires careful selection and making informed choices. This is especially so if you are to avoid the chaotic moments of trying to put something 'quick' together before rushing out to junior's first rugby game.

Here are a few recommended items, which I believe are an essential part of setting you on the right track to creating the occasional healthier meal time. Over time, this would ideally turn out to be a regular occurrence.

Olive Oil.

A good cold pressed, extra virgin olive oil, preferably packaged in a dark bottle (the light weakens the amazing properties in such a phenomenal product). ...."But it's *so* expensive"....I hear you say. Yes, it can be, I agree. That said, if you were to put back a few of the items, especially those of a highly processed and de-natured source, replacing them with just one good quality bottle of the oil aforementioned, then there is no contest.

Balsamic Vinegar.

As with Olive Oil, this is an invaluable ingredient to have in your collection of good food items. This is a wonderful addition to any salad dish when drizzled very sparingly, together with the olive oil. There are variations of infusions when it comes to buying a good salad vinegar, however I would recommend that you can't go wrong by going with a good basic one without several additions on the ingredient list. Pure and simple, I believe, goes a long way when it comes to dressing salads.**

I often find that when baking or roasting veggies, using a drizzle of Balsamic Vinegar can give them a beautiful tang without being overpowering in flavour.

**I remember when I was growing up and 'salad cream' was a delicacy which appeared on special occasions such as when visitors popped in. This was a regular occurrence I might add. Salad Cream was often combined with lettuce and spring onions in a sandwich, and depending on who the visitors were, the sandwich crusts would be carefully removed in order to create a

*good impression. I never did figure out why that was so
important. Was it true that crusts did actually make your
hair go frizzy?*

*It was a happy day when the glass bottle appeared on
the table. If I'd only known then to check the label! Had
I done so, I doubt if I would have been so enthusiastic
about it's appearance amongst our fare. However, I
think there were one or two visitors who were happy to
munch their way through a mighty mound of crustless
sandwiches containing this complex substance,
regardless of its extensive ingredient list.*

Herbs & Spices:

This is something you can build up over time.

I have listed the most commonly used first, so that you
can work your way through the list, adding one every
week or so, depending on what suits your budget.

Of course, as with any ingredient, fresh is always best
and if you have the luxury of growing your own herbs,
then always go for that first.

Cinnamon - Fabulous in taste, versatile in use, and a
great Blood sugar level stabiliser. Cinnamon is an ideal
tool to include for weight loss and those who are
diabetic or who feel they might be at risk of becoming
so. Some of the ways I recommend using Cinnamon
are;-

To sweeten/flavour hot milk.

Sprinkled on top of mashed banana, either served on
warm toast at breakfast, or on rice cakes for afternoon
tea.

A must have baking ingredient in muffins, breads and crumbles.

Combined with other spices in rice dishes.

Sprinkled over porridge or muesli at breakfast.

Sprinkled on top of grated apple, pear or mashed banana mixed with natural yogurt, some oats, a drizzle of honey and a few squashed walnuts, for a super boost after school. (This is a great one to put into a container and bring to the game or practice for in-betweens, but remember to take a spoon!).

Basil - Obviously better freshly picked from the garden, but not always possible. So a good quality dried version can substitute. Basil is a delicious addition to any Italian style dish.
Just in case your long lost Italian cousins show up and you decide to cook for them, I recommend that you hide the dried version until they leave!

Basil, of the fresh variety, is full of vitamins and minerals and is delicious when added to salads or even popped into a sandwich with cheese and tomato or just to nibble at the leaves to help with PMS. I can imagine you all rushing to the nearest neighbour who happens to have an abundance of the fine green leaf and jumping hedges if need be!

Thyme - Fabulous addition to soups and stews. The fresh version chopped very finely and added to pizza topping, thrown into roasts, and pretty much anything else you can imagine on the cooking agenda and as it is not very overpowering, it combines really well with lots of other herbs from the garden.

If that weren't enough, it has lots of vitamins, fibre and minerals to name just a few. Plus it also helps relieve muscle spasms and painful menstrual cycles. I feel you changing gears again in order to stock up on this little all-rounder!

If by now, I have stirred a hidden hunger for education on the properties contained in our flavoursome produce, then I would recommend a book written by *Suzanne Lyle* called *'Eat smart stay well'*. She gives amazing in depth information about everything you could ever wish to know on edible plants.

But for now, I am just 'skirting' the information with an attempt to gear you in the right direction when it comes to everyday choices.

So now that you have stocked up on some of the commonly used herbs, let's not forget the humble salt 'n pepper. Salt gets a lot of bad press, and I believe this is predominantly down to its misuse/over usage and perhaps the wrong 'type' of salt.

If you pick up any food packaged in a tin, a bottle, a jar, a bag or a box, I guarantee almost all will have 'salt' listed on the ingredients. It would be a good idea at this point to begin to familiarise yourself with the possibility of regularly checking the list of ingredients on food items.

More on shopping later, so, for now, just lets stay with the fact that most of our bought food contains salt. You will notice also that those with the most intense flavours, generally contain the most!

So why is salt on the stocking up list?
If I could just get you to swing a little more towards eating a bit fresher. By eating less food which gone through lengthy processing, there remains room to occasionally add a little salt according to your own taste and judgement (personal power) instead of at the mercy of the processing plant.

Other great herbs are;

Black Pepper / Rosemary (which incidentally is grown in abundance every where you look, even around some public pathways!) / Sage / Cumin / Coriander / Chilli / Oregano.
As I mentioned earlier, these can be stocked up on gradually. By doing so, you are more likely to be able to buy the better brands in glass jars which are much cleaner for the pantry and keeps them fresh for longer.

Tomato based products:
Tomato based products are 'heaven sent' in my opinion and I cannot promote them enough. They can be used in any number of ways and come in so many variations.
For starters, the property in tomatoes which gives them their red appearance, just happens to be of incredibly

health giving by protecting our skin from damaging sun rays.

So, here are some of the tomato products which I believe are a 'must have'.

Tomato puree.

This can be found in tins, jars or tubes. I personally would opt for the ones which have nothing else added, just tomatoes and salt.

(as I mentioned earlier, you will find salt added to most processed of foods, so let this be a guideline when it comes to cooking with these products).

Having said that, there is a tomato paste out there which has 'no added salt' on the label so you might want to opt for that one. Great for adding a little to either soups, stews, casseroles, pizza toppings and sauces.

Tinned or Jar Chopped tomatoes.

Again, check on the labels, as there are quite a few of these items containing added sugar as well as lots of other undesirables. I will delve into label reading a little later on, when I navigate you through the supermarket.

Believe it or not, there are lots of varieties available when it comes to tinned tomatoes, (gosh, how exciting can it get!). There are chopped tomatoes with herbs & garlic, chopped tomatoes with herbs, whole peeled tomatoes in tomato juice, in oil & herbs…. the list is endless. My advice would be to choose a variety and be assured that you will call upon them all at some stage. Things I like to use them in are, pasta dishes, salsa, soups, stir fry, ratatouille and sauces.

Tinned, Jar or dried Beans/Peas.

I am not recommending that you predominantly buy and eat out of tins or jars, however when it comes to beans and peas (commonly known as legumes), unless you want to opt for the soaking and longer method of cooking that is necessary with dried legumes, tinned and jar versions are good alternatives. *Ideally the soaking and longer cooking method is superior in quality and overall taste.*

As with the tomato products, check the label and opt for the varieties containing the least amount of added ingredients. Even having chosen the less processed variety, it is still imperative that you empty the contents of the tin into a sieve or colander before cooking, and rinse thoroughly to remove any of the liquid which they have been stored in.

There are numerous ways to use these amazing gatherings of goodness in our meals. First of all there are so many varieties of beans that I would suggest that you get all of them! Mixed, separate, any combination available.

One of my favourite ways to use these is in a pasta mix. With veggies, beans and pasta all in one pan, you have a hearty, nutritious and delicious meal which will satisfy the most picky little eaters.

Other suggestions would be to include beans in stir fry dishes / soups / casseroles / cold in salads / nibble straight from a bowl as a snack.

Nuts & seeds:
Nuts and seeds are often misunderstood, mis represented and for many, they are labelled as either 'bird food' or on their 'bad & forbidden' list.

I have yet to see an overweight and stressed out bird, so that in itself in an incentive to share their liking for the infamous little nibbles.

Simply put, providing you treat nuts and seeds with the respect they deserve, by eating them in their *natural* state, therefore unsalted, unflavoured, un-roasted, unsweetened, un-curried, un *anything*, in *little* portion sizes *staggered throughout the week,* then you can't go wrong. The exception of course is if you have a life threatening allergy to nuts, then caution is advised.

Have you ever had that craving/hunger for something not sweet, not savoury, but just something to nibble on which doesn't resemble a complete meal or snack? The next time this creeps up on you (and it will), reach for Pumpkin Seeds and Cashew Nuts. Not only will you be doing your body a nutritional favour, you will also be putting an end to that mood which was been hanging over you for the past day or so! You *do* know what I'm talking about! Cashew Nuts alone help to release the 'happy hormone' *naturally*.

Today we are very lucky to have such a variety available in our local supermarket, and so well presented that we don't have to search the shelves to find them, nor do we have to buy a kilo at a time.

Be aware if you are thinking about buying nuts or seeds in bulk, they do have a tendency to go a little rancid towards the bottom. I would advise stocking up a little and often. That way, you can spread the cost and there'll be no wastage. Also, because of the high fat content in nuts, they are best stored in glass containers and kept away from light.

Honey
Honey is one of those things where, if you don't already like it then there's enough variations out there to convert you. Lets not forget that just because it's honey and not jam, doesn't mean that you can go wild, spreading a jarful in couple of toast sittings! If you do use honey as a spread on either toast, in a sandwich, under peanut butter in a pita, drizzled on top of yoghurt with or added to hot milk and cinnamon, it's a matter of *how much* that is important.

People have a tendency to think that if they veer towards a 'healthier' product, then it shouldn't matter how much you have. Not so. You can experience the same sugar rush from toast 'laden' with the best quality honey as you would do with sugar laden jam or a piece of candy. So by exercising a little restraint, you will save yourself (and your kids) from sugar highs, whilst benefiting from further stretching the budget.

I will point out that there *are* some ok jams out there on the shelves. However, like everything, read the label, check for undesirables and choose accordingly. If you do opt for your favourite jam in the end, just use it sparingly and it will last for longer.

Peanut Butter / Nut Butter. (such as almond / cashew / brazil)

Peanut Butter is at the heart of much controversy . There seems to be an increasing number of people who are diagnosed as having nut allergies. This is quite tragic as it does mean having to be on the alert for so many things which have nut (traces) tucked away in the bowels of the ingredients list and of course, they are unable to partake in the delicacy of the nut butter. All is not lost however, in that many people who show up as having allergies to nuts are perfectly fine with seeds.

Luckily seed butters are popping up all the time now on the supermarket shelves, such as Tahini (sesame seed paste), Sunflower Butter/Paste and my favourite one of all, Pumpkin Seed paste. Use these alternatives as you would do Peanut/Nut Butters.

Crackers.

This can be where you get creative without too much thought processing. The crackers I would recommend stocking up on are;

Rice Cakes/Corn Thins/ plain Wheat crackers/ old fashioned Oat Cakes.

Again, there are so many varieties available these days, to list them all would take me beyond my deadline for book completion, by which time another few varieties would have crept onto the shelves.

What I would suggest is that you pay attention to the 'flavoured' and 'spiced' and seemingly 'interesting' options, as often times these are laced with salt, artificial

flavourings, preservatives and MSG (which provides the addictive properties in this kind of food item).
The above varieties mentioned may be perceived as boring and/or tasteless, but needn't necessarily be so. There are many ways to include these for 'afternoon tea' or a mid morning snack.

Stocking the Fridge:

The fridge is an area where, the cleaner and simpler it is the better.
Assuming that you have gone through the de cluttering process similar to that of the pantry, the fridge is now clear, clean and awaiting a fine and exciting selection of fresh produce.
No more half-consumed condiments from last year. No more leftover fish pie, which you know in your heart of hearts you would never have re-heated but just didn't have the heart to throw it out.

Milk.

Providing no one in the family has an intolerance, or an adversity to milk, then this is pretty simple. *Organic is best.* I say this with conviction and would recommend making every effort possible to go organic when it comes to dairy products.
Interestingly, research has shown that, in some cases where there was an intolerance to normal milk products, when switched to organic the symptoms seemed to either disappear altogether or lessen somewhat.

This it would seem, is closely linked to the growth hormone which is used for milk production and/or possible addition of antibiotics used for, ironically, 'health maintenance' in dairy cattle. This is not used in organically produced milk.

The same applies to cheese and yoghurt.
I know this sounds idealistic for many and I can hear the shrieks of "I can't afford to go organic on dairy"! so let's explore this a little further.
How much dairy are you consuming at the moment and *in what form?*

The never ending rows of inviting and 'distracting' variations of the simple yoghurt, has gone way beyond what yoghurt was intended for.
If you pick up any one of the kids' yoghurt varieties, you will see a cocktail list of ingredients you really don't want to be feeding your children on a regular basis. Not only are they laced with the infamous sugar, the list goes on to read items which are purposefully targeting the little people's tasted buds and tipping their energy over the edge in a flash!
So how much do *they* cost?
If you were to substitute several 'family packs' of those little tubs, with a big carton or container of 'organic' natural yoghurt, then I guarantee that you would be pleasantly surprised and perhaps on your way to making some permanent changes on your shopping list.

If you are not in favour of Natural Yoghurt by itself, which many aren't, especially kids who have been used to the many flavours that are readily available, it will be necessary to get a little creative and produce your own flavours according to your individual likes and dislikes. After all, no one would expect an immediate request from a six or seven year old to be "Mum can I have a big bowl of organic natural yoghurt?'

Let's start with the idea of the humble mashed banana. Add a drizzle of honey (just a drizzle) and a dusting of cinnamon to jazz it up a little! I really am an advocate of mashed banana. I think this originated from resorting to banana on toast in the absence of inspiration or time and has therefore since become a favourite for myself and for my daughter. Did I tell you how healthy bananas are? They are packed with goodness and can help in a variety of areas such as digestion / constipation *and* diarrhoea, intestinal ulcers and heartburn / morning sickness and are a *natural* antacid. They reduce blood pressure and the risk of stroke. They regulate body water balance and are a great 'hangover' cure. They have a calming effect and can therefore help to improve mood and endure an overall feeling of well being. Obviously due to their relatively high, though natural, fruit sugar content, it's best to keep to a maximum of one per day.

So there you have it! The humble banana not so drab anymore!

Getting back to the yoghurt solution. Other great ways to jazz up the natural yoghurt and make it more palatable for those unfortunate enough not to enjoy it straight, is by adding teaspoonful a spoonful Black strap molasses which is very high in potassium, iron and calcium.

…..My mind wanders to my dear mum's freshly baked treacle bread…..

By adding any of your favourite fruit or berries, either raw or cooked, you can create your own version of flavoured yoghurt without the list of undesirable ingredients.

You can see how simple it is to create a mouth watering, healthy, nutritious and economical alternative to those confusing packages on the shelves. Any of these suggestions can be transferred into a small pot, spoon in hand and straight into the school lunchbox!

Cheese.
The cheese counter can be just as confusing, with flavours, 'bits' added and the 'spreadable' versions. The same applies as does for the yoghurts in the sense that, the purer and plainer the better. There appears to be a lot of hype about the high fat and cholesterol content in cheese and therefore many people feel that the option for them, if they are to improve their health, would be to opt for the 'low fat' or the 'fat free' option. *More later about the clever marketing which draws us to the 'low fat' promise during Supermarket shopping.*

As per the other dairy items mentioned earlier, choosing a 'low fat' or 'fat free' version will neither satisfy your taste buds, or help you on your way to a smaller waistline. Surprised? What you will find is this. As the fat is removed, it is firmly replaced with copious amounts of sugar/sugar substitutes/favouring and 'enhancers'.
Our brain actually *needs* fat in order to function optimally. So unless you are seriously intolerant to dairy,

I would include it in your intake and perhaps reduce the quantity and *frequency* eaten.

And now to the **daily spread**!
Do you choose butter? or do you choose margarine for it's convenience, price, popularity and spreadability? A loaded question indeed! Going on nature alone, I would of course recommend butter. It has gone through less processing and is therefore more natural than it's artificial impostor.

As with all items previously mentioned, a little goes a long way and if it's a budgeting decision that prompts you to choose margarine over butter, I urge you to reconsider and explore including introducing some of the nut and seed spread options mentioned earlier on.

3. Navigating the Supermarket.

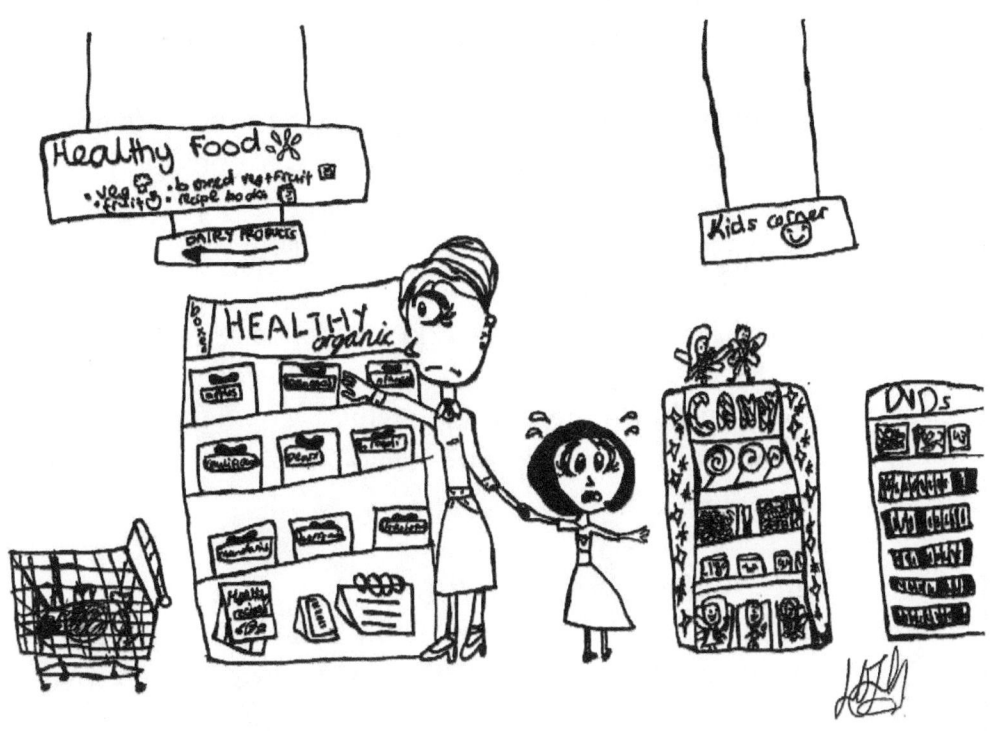

There are a few guidelines I would like to offer that will help you to turn what is often perceived as anything from mundane, to downright frustrating and hellish, into a successful, economical and easy weekly venture.
I am not insinuating that everyone dreads the weekly shop. Some may find it a delightful experience, therefore spending hours just pondering the shelves, floating from aisle to aisle, with an endorphin rush having spotted the newest item on the shelf since last

visit. If this describes you, you may want to consider becoming a professional personal shopper? ...just a thought.

The 'dos' and the 'don'ts';
1. Always make a shopping list. (and remember to bring the list with you!)
2. If at all possible, do the shopping when the kids are at school or alternatively, when they are being looked after.
3. Always make sure your tummy isn't running on empty when you shop.
4. Get to know your supermarket and where everything is.
5. Shop mainly on the outside aisles
6. Be conscious of marketing tricks.
7. Get in. Get out, Done!

1. Always make a shopping list.
Ensure you actually have your list at hand when you go into the supermarket, and use it. If you shop from a plan, you are much less likely to fall into the hands of the visual stimulants. By this I mean, you will not tempted to get what *looks* nice but don't actually need (the impulse buy). By following this guideline, your weekly shopping actually results in being much less expensive in the long run.

2. Shop without the kids if possible.
We've all been there, trying to divert the hands of a little one, who is desperately trying to add one or two items from the multitude of 'strategically placed' candy, into

the trolley, or directly into their tummy. You just don't need this additional stress.

The conflict arises when not wanting to appear to be the Mother from hell by yanking your child from their pleasure quest and dragging, if necessary, to accompany you on the rest of your shopping journey.

The alternative 'unthinkable' is taking the path of avoiding further protest by giving in to the plea for an instant sugar hit! The latter though does have a tendency to come back and bite you. The after effects of the aforementioned, tend to make an appearance before the shopping is complete.

I do realise that it is not always possible to go it alone, so what I would suggest for the little ones who need to come with you, is to bring their favourite, 'quiet', engrossing and time-consuming toy/educational item along for the ride. It's never too young to start working with the infamous Rubix Cube! This is exactly when the 'list' is needed most.

3. *Always make sure your tummy isn't running on empty when you enter the sliding doors!*

This is one I have personally had many challenges with in the past. I would often head out on one of my runs, bringing my cash card (& possibly a little list of the very few things I needed to pick up on my way home, which I could carry in a light bag in each hand as I ran). I want to stress here that, whether you are a seasoned runner or just a very busy Mum (obviously nothing wrong with being both!), you will recognise that when hunger sets in after running, no time is spent on checking labels, waiting until you are home and have had your shower, or in fact, waiting until you leave the supermarket! It was those times in particular that even the meat counter of the deli section could entice the most 'vegan' of vegetarians! For the running Mums out there, you know what I'm talking about….. your tummy is growling, your head's a little 'spacey', you're getting irritable with the lady who just won't move her trolley and you're on a mission of satisfy that need for edible, anything will do! The list goes further into your pocket and your eyes do the 'walking'.

It is fascinating how your taste buds are stimulated so tangibly when you glide your gaze over the snack section when you are hungry.
You unwittingly reach out for the 'snack'n dips'. None of which you would ordinarily have the incline for, but right now, you couldn't imagine there to be a more satisfying gastronomic experience. So, you reach for the kill, vowing to return to healthier options once the packet is empty.

4. *Know the layout of the supermarket*
Have you ever been thrown into confusion after returning from holiday, by popping into your local supermarket to pick up some basic items and finding yourself an hour later still trying to figure out where anything is?
I would imagine, given that we are generally quite habitual beings, the tendency is to do the weekly shop in the same supermarket each time.
This is where it pays to have a good mental picture of where to find your listed items. In fact, I would go one step further in saying that it might pay to structure your list according to the layout of the supermarket.

I am at risk here of exposing myself as a complete fruit cake, with a need to get a life outside of shopping, but if my eccentricities can help, then it's truly worth it.

Even though it may sound just a little above and beyond the call of a weekly shop, from personal experience, this little exercise saves time, frustration and unwanted items, plus it gets the job done with the utmost efficiency.

5. *Shop mainly in the outside aisles.*

I hear many of you saying "That's where the wine is!" The majority of the outside aisles are chilled. Chilled aisles contain items which are on the 'fresher' end of the spectrum.

An example of this would be the difference between 'milk from the chilled section' and the 'long life' variety found in the middle aisles.

The long life variety can withstand the temperatures of regular surroundings and can sit on the shelf for a matter of months, maybe longer. Compare that to milk found in the chilled section where there is a definite expiry date, which is probably no longer than a few days from display.

So given this sort of evidence, it's pretty easy to have guess which contains the undesirable ingredients necessary to create the long lasting properties of the product.

The fresh fruits and vegetables, herbs and salads, do take centre stage in the outer aisles it would be advisable to remain in this section for as long as possible.

Having advised you to concentrate on the outer aisles, they can also throw some challenges your way.
The dairy section, as I may have uttered some sentiments about previously, can be a tricky one to navigate. Not only are there way too many choices, many also contain more than basic milk ingredients. Many yoghurts contain equal amounts, and sometimes more, sugar than an average scoop of ice cream.
What about juices? I could dedicate a whole chapter alone on juices and their pros and cons.

If you think about how juice is made, fruit juice such as the popular Orange Juice that routinely appears on the average breakfast table.
How many oranges do you think it takes to make the average glass of the orange juice. Approximately six to eight! I don't know about you, but doubt if I would have the capacity to munch my way through six or eight oranges *before* eating breakfast. And I can assure you I have a pretty healthy sized appetite, *especially* for breakfast. But technically speaking, that is what you would be consuming in sugar content and in energy value (calories).
All the above *without* the goodness of the fleshy bits. This refers to the fruit juices that *don't* have sugar added, so imagine what the *added* sugar varieties will do to your blood sugar levels! So again, a little 'label checking' is always advised.
My message here is not to steer you away from one of the most popular morning starters but to create a little awareness and encourage you to occasionally choose to eat the whole fruit instead.

6. *Be conscious of marketing tricks!*

You and I, no doubt at some point in our shopping experiences, have fallen into the trap of being won over by clever marketing strategies. Mistakenly believing that we were either making a positive financial decision that will save us countless dollars, or buying the ultimate product that promises to change our lives forever! If only that were true....

Supermarkets, and the same applies to any retail business within our reach, are pretty clever when it comes to creating a desire or a 'need'. The downfall there is, if you are not conscious of the *intent* of the displays, packaging or promises laid out, it is easy to find justification for every unnecessary purchase. From packets of the latest variety of the '*nutty omega wonder breakfast cereal*' or the face cream which will '*melt away those signs of ageing in just 2 weeks*' to the promise of your children never having to go to the dentist again as a result of the latest '*enriched with calcium*' snack item on the shelves.
 So I reiterate the importance of a shopping list and sticking to it.

7. *Get in and Get out!*

Enter the supermarket, list at hand, do your shopping at a rate of knots and get out of there as if your pants were on fire!
I really believe that the more time you have to do something, the more time it takes for you to do it.
Have you noticed that when you have a multitude of various after school activities (especially those who have more than one child in the family, each one with a

different venue to attend), that you often get things done and done on time?

As per the familiar quote "If you want something done, give it to a busy person".

The chances are, that you also squeezed in a supermarket trip mid schedule and if so, time is of the essence.

Just incase you are blessed with time abundant days of blissful self expression, freedom and void of pressure beyond deciding where to eat lunch, it might be worth *inventing* a busy schedule. A busy schedule could prompt you in adhering to the 'get in and get out' mindset and avoid unnecessary impulse buys in the process!

4. What are People Eating Today?

A low down on what people are actually eating on any given day.

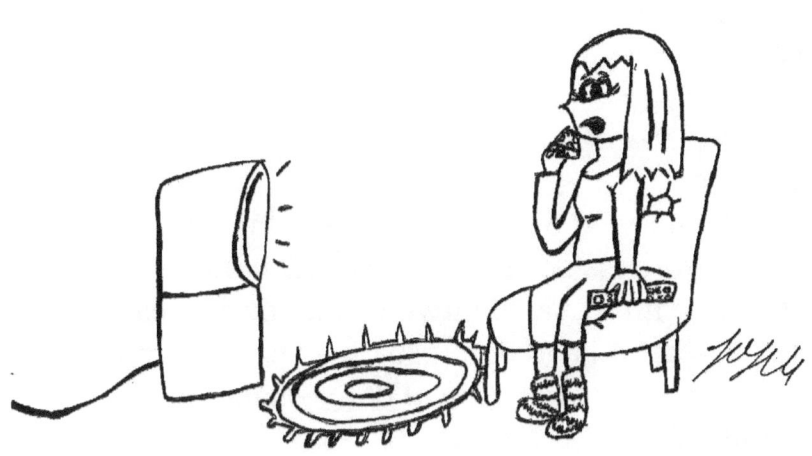

I have always been fascinated to observe the eating habits of our fellow humans. We scurry our way through our busy lives, often reaching for what is available at the time, and sometimes with the thought that 'no one is watching'.

Whether you are on 'big brother' while you eat, or having a quiet private moment to nourish the engine and replenish the soul, what matters most is *how well* you are fuelling your miraculous make up that is your body.

In my curiosity into the minor details of what people are really eating in a typical day, I was given the privilege to take a deeper look at how a few selected individuals fuelled their engines on a regular basis.

This by no means represents the nation as a whole, but I felt that it would give me a little insight into what some individual choices are and more interestingly, how their health & wellbeing is as a whole .

My three subjects are as follows;
1.
Michelle is a 43 year old self-proclaimed insomniac, carrying a few dress sizes more than she would like. She is a single mum, raising two boys, one 13 year old and one 10 year old and doing so on a very low budget. When I had a look at her typical daily intake, the first thing I noticed quite prominently was *tea*! Lots of it! Sarah drinks a minimum of 10 cups of tea with skimmed milk, on a daily basis. The remainder of her consumption of food and beverages consists of the following:

Porridge / Vegemite sandwich on multigrain bread / Banana / '2 minute' noodles with vegetables, cooked in soy oil & soy sauce / Large instant coffee made with milk and water with sugar added.
Although this does not represent *every* day, the correlation between disrupted sleep patterns and the

consumption of caffeinated beverages seems to be relatively obvious.

What is also evident, is the correlation between overall *low caloric* intake and the resistance to weight loss. As I am sure by now, the evidence of the 'low calorie intake' and difficult weight management is widely known and understood. However, for the benefit of those who are still in any doubt, **a low calorie intake** (ie lower than the average recommended for gender, age and height) **on a *consistent* basis and for *extended periods of time*, is not the path to a smaller dress size**. Whilst dramatically reducing your daily intake may *initially* give way to some weight loss, it will very quickly return plus a few extra pounds, on resuming normal consumption, unless of course there are major alterations in lifestyle in the process.

According to Michelle, the low calorie intake is unintentional. Given Michelle's budget and busy life raising her boys, 'diet' is far from her list of priorities. I commend her for her resourcefulness when it comes to home grown produce, which is in abundance in the confines of her back yard. This in itself is an inspiration for anyone on a low budget who feels they cannot afford to eat healthily.

So where can she shift a few things around to address the sleep issues and perhaps loose a few pounds in the process, *plus* stay within her budget?

The first thing I would address is the tea issue. There's absolutely nothing wrong with the occasional cup of tea and very often it's just the ticket when in need of a little comfort, relaxation, an engine boost or a simple 'tea and banter with your nearest and dearest'.

In Michelle's case, the tea issue is more a combination of a crutch and a habit.

What I would suggest to anyone wanting to cut back on any habit such as tea (or coffee), is to make very *small, subtle* adjustments on a *consistent* basis.

For example, for the first week, substitute one or two cups of tea with either a glass water with a slice of lemon or lime, or alternatively hot water with freshly picked mint leaves or freshly grated ginger (great for digestion). Then progressively, week by week, replace one more cup with an alternative until the tea consumption is reduced to a level where it no longer has the disrupting effect on sleep patterns or categorised as an 'addiction'.

The issue of Michelle's low caloric intake could easily be rectified by replacing for example, the 'two minute noodles' or the 'instant coffee made with skimmed milk and sugar', with a nutritious, filling and economical smoothie. By getting rid of the highly processed and often expensive packaged 'ready in two minutes' meal, it will reduce the toxic overload that contributes to resistance in weight loss. It will nourish her body with 'real' food and bump up her overall caloric intake, As well as providing her with additional savings on her shopping bill.

An example suggestion for the smoothie would include, though not exclusive to;

Full fat Milk / Banana / Home grown in-season berries or substitute which can be plucked from her back yard / Handful of nuts or seeds.

A good winter alternative could be; Soup consisting of vegetables in season, with the addition of legumes.

These simple additions and substitutions to Michelle's daily intake would generously bring her calorie intake to a healthier level, gradually alleviate her sleep disruptions and in the process, give her metabolic rate a boost. (*more on metabolism later.*)

The way to create long lasting change in any pattern/ habit, is to do so very *gradually* and very *subtly*. This way the body doesn't overtly detect the changes made, but *over time*, can transform an unhealthy habit into a health giving practice.

2.
The second individual I interrogated was Sue, a 57 year old retiree who had just discovered the gym, having lost the equivalent in kilos of her shadow self after diligent working on a 'points' system of 'dieting'. I have to tread a little carefully here, as I have the potential to be rather judgemental about anything that requires a regimented ritual of converting food into points and judging whether you are 'good' or 'bad' according to what the 'weigh in' reads.

Within this kind of strategy, you would also be 'rewarded' for, what could be the result of wearing different clothing, the time of the month, the temperature, or the fact that you may not be wearing your chunky necklace when stepping on the fluctuating machine that lies under your trembling feet.
Let's just have a look at what a typical day of 'point scoring' looks like for Sue:

Breakfast; consisting of half a banana (what happens to the other half?), a kiwi fruit, 1lb tub of greek yoghurt, 2 slices of wholemeal bread with honey and tea with added 'trim' milk. This comes to a total of *6 points*! This exercise in itself is an added maths task you hadn't plan for since leaving college.

Sue's breakfast as it stands, would appear to be pretty ideal for most people.

There's a cup of tea thrown in the mix a little later on in the morning, followed by lunch consisting of either a bagel or 2 slices of toast. Toppings would consist of hummus or tuna with a little salad on the side. There's even a touch of mayonnaise in there too! All this adds up to *4 points*, including another cup of tea. Again, it sounds like relatively healthy options (apart from the mayonnaise, although *if used sparingly and infrequently*, it would not necessarily create a life or death scenario).

Mid afternoon Sue's afternoon 'treat' consists of a carefully measured - points counted - system friendly -'health bar' (and I use the word 'health' loosely) with a cup of tea. All of which, tallies to another *1 and a half to 2 points*. For something that is so small and takes but a slight inhale to consume, it doesn't seem fair to expend any points on this.

I did investigate the ingredient list on the package of the 'health bar' and my findings were no surprise. Although low in fat content, which I mentioned earlier was not necessarily a good thing, it contained enough sugar and sugar giving ingredients in there to seriously spike blood sugar levels. ***Any foods containing either corn syrup or high fructose corn syrup are contenders for***

***contributing to excess belly fat and ultimately the risk
of diabetes.***

The infamous promise of the 'Diet Bar', the 'Low fat
loose 5 kilos while you eat it' bar continues. I reiterate
my guidelines for avoiding clever marketing strategies
mentioned in the previous chapter.

*Back in the 70s and 80s and up until her last breath, my
dear Mum was always taken in by the enticing diet and
weight loss trends. She embarked on many regimes in a
bid to lose weight (and I have to add, sometimes did, but
always gained it back and more!). The thing I recall
most about her quest to lose weight, was that she would
buy crackers which had the promise to 'bring your
waistline in line with that of Bo Derek, (for those who
are too young to remember Bo Derek, just think Scarlet
Johansen or the likes). Mum would eat her normal meal
of 'meat and two veggies accompanied with perhaps a
helping of ice cream' and then have her cracker in the
hope it would do it's magic. I guess she never did grasp
the 'replacement' idea.   ………… I digress..*

Dinner for Sue is a simple Baked Potato with a
vegetable stir fry (in a carefully measured teaspoonful of
oil) and a little soy sauce. Followed by a tea and a
sneaky 'bar' as per above! All that for *3 points*.
Sue summed this particular day up as a 'Good Day', a
'low points day'.
I don't know about you, but when I think of the mental
energy and the pressure to 'be good' is combined in a

frantic calculating guilt trip, I doubt if I would be a compliant candidate for such an arrangement.

I guess by now you have figured out that I am not a huge fan of this sort of regimental daily confinement.

What I *would* add, is that there are several reasons why this kind of system seems to work for so many (all-be-it for some, very temporarily).

Firstly, the *accountability* which is necessary when having to show up and 'weigh in' coupled by the sheer humiliation of 'not doing it' and therefore being a 'very bad person indeed', is enough motivation to stick rigidly to any given instructions.   There is also of course, the group support. Evidently, whenever a group is formed for a purpose such as 'weight loss', the motivation to succeed often stems from the secret competition between new best mates. There is also the additional group support and encouragement which go hand in hand with common goals, especially challenging goals.

It probably sounds like I am having a change of heart regarding the 'meeting and weighing in' idea, rest assured I am not. I still believe that there are gentler paths to take in order to drop a dress size.

Let's look at a few strategies that are incorporated in programs like this, without the regimented number crunching.

One successful component of a program like this is the accountability given and received amongst the participants. Accountability can easily be attained by choosing an accountability partner for yourself. Choose someone who *will* hold you accountable, at all times.

You know the type of person I am referring to, the person you would never want to catch you in your

onesie, curled up in front of the TV slurping your way through your second helping of chocolate frozen yoghurt!
Make it known to them that you are making some lifestyle changes and rest assured you will be 'checked up on' or asked "how's the new regime going?" on a regular basis.

The group idea? This can be as equally economic. Gather together a couple of your friends, arrange to take a regular hike together, a regular game of communally enjoyed team sport, a swim, or anything else which will get you moving. The result? group support! People who will hopefully not make you feel like a 'really bad person' for not living up to the mark, and as a bonus, you're likely to have some fun too.

3.
The following individual is one who fascinates me. As well as providing me with a glimpse into some of the food trends of our next generation, it gives an indication of how food and energy can play a huge role in school performance and development.

Francesca is a busy fifteen year old college student and dancer, who also plays a role teaching dance to some of the younger kids.

Francesca puts her heart and soul into her dance, and often school work fits in around her dance schedule. In addition, she is often challenged at school, having been diagnosed as dyslexic.

I have to say, as a teenager, Francesca is an incredibly likeable, fun loving and genuinely good hearted young individual, who I believe has a bright future in the dance and performing arts world.

I would however recommend that she make some serious changes around her food choices, before it starts to catch up with her.

Here's why:

Francesca starts her day 'on the run', apple in hand which has to keep her going until her 10am break, when she grabs a muesli bar, yes, one of the 'health bars' I mentioned earlier.

She resists the temptation to reach for more than one bar at a time, which I do applaud her for, given that they usually come in boxes of six or eight and once opened it can be difficult to exercise restraint. However, sticking to just one leaves her vulnerable to the temptation of the 'spider lollies' from the school canteen at her 11.30am interval. This is often alternated with a cookie (the packaged ones with the cute smiley face on the front!).

12.20pm rolls around and *Chocolate* is imminent. Balanced only by the piece of fruit brought from home. (Mum smiles when she sees the fruit going into the bag, oblivious to the dark recesses of the canteen temptations!).

A bag of chips is Francesca's dessert washed down with a can of ......dare I even say it......*Soda* (liquid sugar combined with added chemical cocktail).

The already consumed cocktail of sugar, preservatives, colouring, and depending on the soda, added caffeine, has no doubt taken it's toll on Francesca's concentration, leaving her tired, irritated and her body crying out for 'real food'.

Luckily Francesca has no choice but to give in to the calling of her nutritionally depleted body at around 3.30pm. Back in the vicinity of her Mum again, she munches her way through some fresh pineapple, a banana, some cheese and a few wholemeal crackers, washed down with a glass of fresh milk and followed by an apple.

The evening meal is generally a balanced home cooked ensemble and often polished off with a helping of vanilla ice cream. (Perfectly acceptable if that were the only smidgen of decadence for the day, though unfortunately, that's not the case here).

Evening is topped with another piece of fruit and a cup of tea.

Given the sequence and content of consumption up until coming home from school, it doesn't take a Scientist, Nutritionist, or a Physician to suspect a correlation between school performance, general motivation in a learning environment and what goes into the body to nourish/fuel it.

My guess is that Francesca is by no means alone in her food choices on any given day, especially within her peers, and environment in general.

If Francesca were to alter, *even a few,* of her early morning to lunch time choices, she would experience a significant shift in energy, motivation, learning ability, focus and overall feeling of wellbeing.

I have absolutely no doubt in my conviction with this. The only stumbling block there may be, is the resistance to change and the initial 'withdrawal' of sugar and highly processed food.

In my chapter on 'Suggested recipes', some of the breakfast options would ideally provide Francesca with the nutritional fuel necessary in order to take on any challenge a learning environment may provide.

So having had a look at a *minuscule* section of the general public and their eating habits, it would be fair to say, that changing even just one or two food options *on a consistent basis, over time*, would result in a giant leap for sustained health and well being.

BY TAKING SMALL STEPS NOW, YOU WILL BE TAKING A GIANT LEAP FOR YOUR FUTURE

..............Since beginning writing this chapter, Sue, my subject number 2, now in her sixties, gave up her 'weekly weigh ins' and instead started making a few simple food and lifestyle changes **on a consistent basis.** *She now enjoys living life on her own terms, with a newfound vibrance likened to that of a thirty year old. She has also started a new career teaching and inspiring young media students. She loves the freedom which accompanies vibrant and sustained health, and as a positive side effect, has effortlessly dropped a couple of dress sizes in the process!*

....

5. The Baking Revolution.

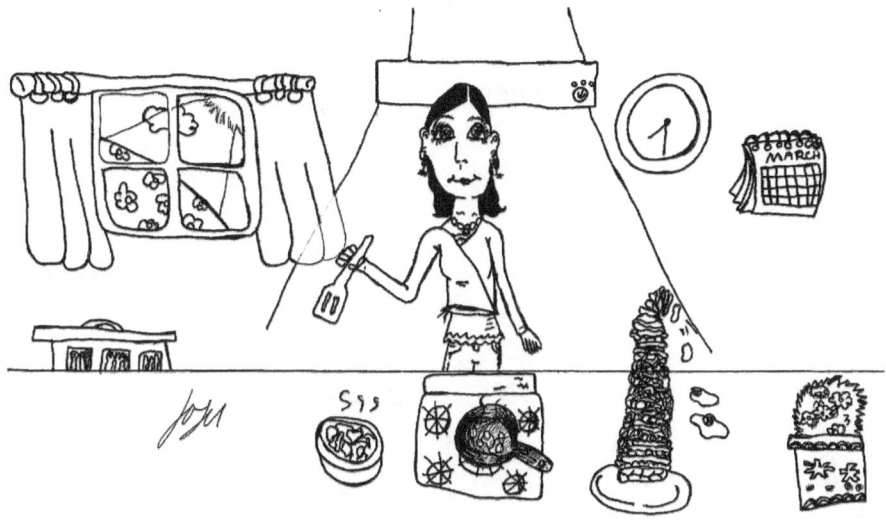

When I first moved her to New Zealand I was struck, and impressed by, the amount of baking which took place in the average household on a regular basis. From brownies, to quiches, from scones to cookies, from cup cakes to full blown iced cakes. I never imagined that I too would succumb to the lure of the hot oven!
I had quite arrogantly slotted baking into a category for those who had 'nothing better to do' and who had small children who needed entertaining in the form of sticky fingers! Admittedly, I also blamed a lot of the baking culture for the increase in jean sizes worn by those standing in the kitchen, sweat pouring, hovering over the next batch of perfectly risen double chocolate-chocolate chip muffins.

So why have I too, succumbed to the lure of the freshly baked? Well, baking and I go back a long way and I guess I have rekindled a kind of passion which I had pushed aside in a bid to be super healthy. I was oblivious to the ideal scenario of possibly staying healthy *and* enjoying occasional baking (having your cake *and* eating it), providing you know how.

I have the fondest memories of Mum on Saturday nights, tupperware containers at the ready for the tumultuous mounds of cup cakes, flans, soda bread, treacle bread and the occasional apple or rhubarb tart. Cup cakes didn't have the flash 'cup cake' label then, they were just 'buns' and sometimes, time permitting, became 'iced buns'. The quantity baked, frequently ran into the 60s and beyond.

After all, I did come from a family of 7 kids, Mum & Dad, and Great Aunt Maggie, who lived with us on the farm. The relentless stream of cousins, aunts & uncles, friends and neighbours, never perfected the art of 'making arrangements' to visit. They frequently 'showed up' at will, testimony to Mum's readily available hospitality. On those occasions it was imperative, and I would go as far as to liken it to a religion, that buns were constantly at the ready.

I watched on, observing and mesmerised by the sheer speed at which the production of baked goods would take place, all without a cookbook in sight.

It was a race to scrape the bowl out and lick every last drop of, yes, raw cake mix, before the bowl would be lined up again for yet another batch of delicacies.
I can now understand how the frequent stomach cramps, lethargy and bouts of nausea were linked to this practice. I guess there was less investigation into the occasional tummy troubles then, and more of the 'Eat up' 'Clean up' and 'Get out of my way' kind of scenario'. (I do not condone the practice of eating raw cake mix, or the dismissal of small children in such a manner).

Mum always did the best she knew how, with the knowledge she had at the time.

The whole baking experience didn't go without the incredible valuable lessons which I carry with me to this day. Lessons such as improvising on 'standard' recipes and using substitute ingredients that result in being a lot kinder to the waistline.

I carry the legendary 'trial and error' when it comes to 'how much' and 'what' ingredients to use and the results, more often than not, make me smile.

So where are the 'pitfalls of baking' we very often fall prey to?

1. The little 'end' pieces.
Let's examine for example, the process of baking a simple batch of cookies. Whether chocolate, raisin, shortbread, peanut or coconut.

Have you noticed the somewhat 'insignificant little end piece' of mixture left in the bowl?

In the absence of a young child from back in the late sixties, who would deal with the leftover mixture in one lick of the spoon, the only thing left to do is to pop it onto the tray in a bid to turn it into the 'trial' one when they come out of the oven.

There it is! your first vulnerability, either for yourself or for the little eyes hovering over the 'tail ends'. Why make such a fuss over something so trivial, and on the face of it, really wouldn't do much harm? If this occurs *consistently,* then *over time*, this can become habit forming, and an easily overlooked part of your total daily food consumption.

Just because it isn't necessarily viewed as a whole cookie, it doesn't take away the fact that it has been made to the same formula, therefore contains exactly the same in terms of fat, sugar and energy/calories, and will go in exactly the same direction as the other cookies which are consumed as 'cookies'.

It is advised to exercise a little vigilance around potential 'unconscious' consumption. (more about consciousness later).

My advice therefore, is to have the tupperware container, or similar, at the ready. Then, as soon as those little mouthfuls of pure deliciousness are cool enough, put them in the freezer. Yes, all of them!

Later, when you feel the 'urge' for something to nibble on, especially when your favourite soap is on TV, there should be enough 'thawing' time to really ask yourself the question, "do I really need this right now or could I settle for a 'cuppa' instead?".

I do recall times when the 'frozen muffin' did look inviting and was easily attacked with a sharp implement or held over a warm kettle (I don't have a microwave in my kitchen)! And that's ok! as long as it doesn't become a *habit* which could be difficult to let go of.

Pitfall number 2. Sticking rigidly to the recipe.

I'm guessing we all have them, lurking in the kitchen cupboard, taking pride of place on the open kitchen book shelves, in the allocated kitchen drawer or sitting prominently on the kitchen workbench. I'm referring to recipe books, cup cake books, baking books, loose sheets of paper ripped out of magazines from the Dr's waiting room(not condoning theft!), or printouts of recipes from recent reality TV cooking series.

But who said you had to keep to the letter? What's the worst thing that could happen if you wandered off the beaten track of the list of given ingredients? Chances are you could create something even more amazing! I have learned some important lessons through experimentation and from really wanting to enjoy the delicious home baked goodies, *without* the added dread of an expanding waistline. I realised that whilst it is probably necessary to have one or two recommended basic ingredients in the recipe, the remaining ingredients can be left to your imagination, taste preference and according to what is available in your pantry at the time of baking.

We are so lucky today to have such an array of options which when substituting with, can turn a 'heart attack waiting to happen' into 'a guilt free gastronomic delight'.

Pitfall number 3. When 'tasting' becomes overindulgence.
This pitfall is one that I fondly remember succumbing to with my mum.

One of Mum's most spectacular dishes was creamy rice pudding. It was best to make this dish in a generously sized casserole, as it would allow for slow, deliberate, unadulterated brilliance in the oven, as well as providing enough for all the family to eat.

When the dish was complete, it was placed on the table to allow it to cool before being 'stored for later consumption' ……..it occasionally didn't reach the point of storage…..

Always having been a nibbler, Mum would have the first taste, straight from the casserole. Seconds later, I was ushered to get myself a spoon and give it a try too. I never hesitated. I too sunk my spoon into the scalding spectacle of creamy deliciousness.
Once the tasting began, there was no going back. Mum sitting at one end of the casserole, me at the other. I was in heaven and judging by what was left in the dish, as was my Mother!

I am not suggesting that this is a green light for either greed, or over consumption. What I *would* recommend is this. Firstly, some of the ingredients which were used back then, could very easily be 'tweaked'. Substituting for example, the high sugar content with alternatives such as fruit/cinnamon/a *little* raw sugar or a *little* maple syrup.

Secondly, if you need to 'have a taste' (just to check whether it is palatable enough to serve others), then do just that, have a *taste* not the whole thing. Portion it out according to how many are going to be consuming it and the rest goes in the freezer. Out of sight.

Ultimately I am an advocate of home baking, though some thought needs to go into making it a 'health giving' experience, as well as a thoroughly enjoyable creation that can be passed down from generation to generation. Regarding the latter, things are always evolving and growing, as does revelations in health and how we can become ambassadors of a healthy nation. So endeavour to pass on on trends which are going to *support* your children in living long, happy and healthy lives.

6. Move it! .....you know you can.

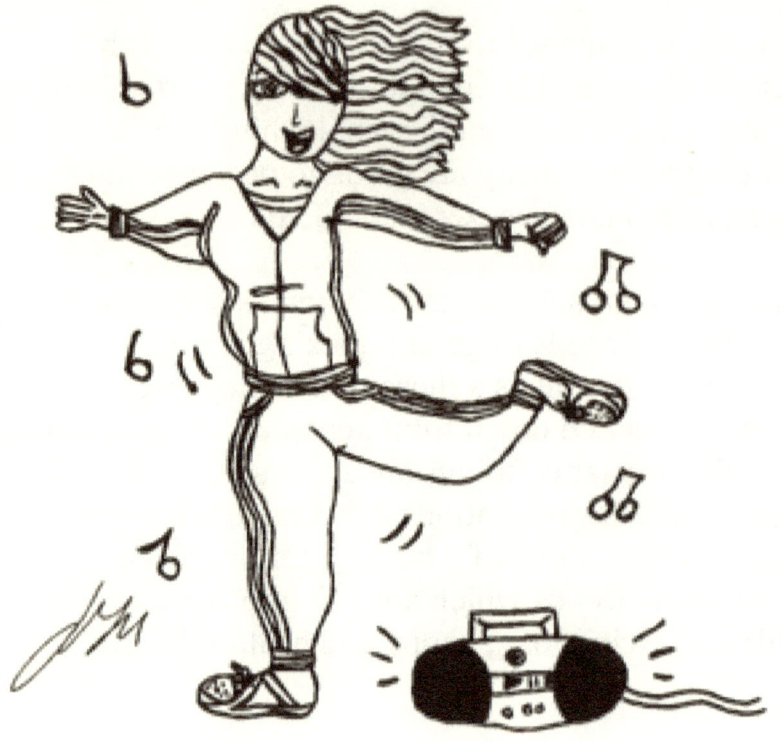

How many times have you heard the sentiments " I *used* to be quite fit" or "I *used* to be a runner but I can't run any more because of my knees" or "my back"....? Have you perhaps muttered something similar yourself?

What would your response be to the question - 'Are you able to successfully get out of bed in the morning by yourself?' If the answer is 'yes', then this tells me that you have the ability to physically make movement with your body, at some level.

Unless you are permanently bedridden, without the ability to move, unassisted, to the extent that you need someone to hold this book and turn the pages for you, then it is possible to move your body *gradually* towards the health which is your birthright.

My apologies for sounding a little harsh here, but people often fall into the 'excuse trap' and it is therefore my intention to bring a little glimmer of hope and possibility to those who would ordinarily spiral down the sedentary path.

Reflecting on days gone by, have you noticed when you look back on some photos of yourself from one or two decades ago, or watched some revival of the 70's TV shows, people in general (self included) appeared to be on the 'lighter' side of the scale? Of course this is not a sweeping representation, but it would be fair to say that it is true for many.

How has this happened? What has occurred in the years in between?

Giving an educated guess, I would say more than likely that *habits* were formed, which when carried out *on a consistent basis over time*, formed the results which people are now trying desperately to correct in record time.

One example of how things have changed, all-be-it something very trivial, is with the introduction of the TV remote control.

For those of you reading this who are too young to remember life without the remote control, let me outline what it actually involved.

I can't relay about 'surfing channels' then as in our household at least, there was one person in charge of what we all watched and that was generally a parent. Perhaps not so for everyone.

Getting back to the art of channel changing. Changing the channel required a conscious effort to use the biggest muscle group, that of those in the buttocks and legs, to assert the position for standing from seated position (from a possible 'slouch' on the sofa), contracting the 'core muscles' (abdominals and lower back), moving through what is now called in fitness terms a 'squat', to either a forward reach or a walk in the direction of the TV set. The length of walk or reach depended upon on how far the sofa was positioned from the TV.

When now positioned in front of the TV, an exerted effort to push the channel button was required. Perhaps a few times until satisfied with the chosen program, in which case the half forwards reach was static and therefore used exerted effort in the buttocks and legs. The retreating effort was executed in a backwards lunge to take up the seated or slouching position previously held, but with a renewed circulatory benefit and a refreshed oxygenated brain.

Compare that to the quick and non exerted effort of the mere thumb press of today!

This is just one example of many, where inventions such as washing machines, microwaves and mobile phones, have resulted in a much more sedentary existence.

Enough delving into the archives, as I believe by now you hear my message.

People in general just aren't moving throughout the day like they did some years ago.

Whilst it is commendable to do your quota of exertion in the gym, do you really need to drive there? You may even cut your time in half if you were to jump on your bike and cycle, or walk/jog to the gym. Once there, spend a concentrated effort in the equipment/weights section followed by a return bike/walk-jog.

By taking this approach, you also avoid lining up for the showers, waisting time gossiping in the locker room midst the shuffling of exposed dressing and undressing. (I guess my catholic heritage just likes to reserve a little dignity when it comes to undressing!).

Let's look at some routine chores that have evolved over time, not always for the better. How many people today hire a cleaner? Vacuuming is personally a task that I continue to have a love/hate relationship with.

Inserting the winter duvet inside a freshly laundered cover is another. (Surely there must be someone out there who could invent an appliance to make the latter task a little less frustrating!)

I can clearly see however, how much of a sweat can be worked up by dragging the vacuum cleaner around, pushing and pulling, moving furniture out of the way, resulting in the entire activity being a great energy expending exercise.

I doubt if I would actually want to hire someone to do this for me, giving up my regular bonus workout that results in my house looking ship shape. Win win!!

Simply put, if you were to incorporate *some* extra moving into you day, in whatever shape or form, *over time* it will create huge payoffs in the energy you have and the 'feel-good' factor you enjoy. It will also offer a reduction in your doctor's bills *and* increase how great you look in (and out of) your clothes. As a ripple effect, the more people benefit from the above experiences, the happier they become.

Given our unique individuality, I will not design a *specific* fitness program for you to follow. Even though there are a lot of similarities between various individuals, your actual body dynamics and requirements are very unique to you.
If you have not been actively involved in any form of fitness up until now and plan to undertake a scheduled fitness program, take it *slowly* at first and commit to it for the long haul.
Fitness is like a puppy, it's not just for Christmas - it's for life!
In order to figure out what type of fitness/activity is suitable for you, give some thought to the following;

Schedule only that which you can commit to no matter what. By doing this, it leaves little room for proverbial excuse to kick in.
Consider it like brushing your teeth. When on vacation, are you likely to stop brushing your teeth? Maintaining some form of physical activity, even when situations and environments change, will result in your physical state resembling that of a well-oiled machine. Commitment and determination doesn't take up luggage space!

Find an activity that you enjoy.
**In the words *Carl Jung....* "*What did you do as a child that would make the hours pass like minutes? Therein lies the key to your earthly pursuits*"*.....*

This is vitally important if you are going to maintain life long physical activity.

If you absolutely hate to run you are not alone. There are many people who feel that running is only necessary if you need to catch a bus and are a little late, or running away from a stray dog on your heels. If this describes you, then I would not recommend starting a fitness program involving running.

Likewise, if you've never really enjoyed team sports or group activities, you are more likely to opt for the more solitary type activities which you will maintain for the long term.

A great way to figure out what kind of activities really hits the spot with you, is to recall your childhood at the age of 7 or 8 years old. **What kind of activity gave you joy? What kind of activity did you do *without* having to be coerced by persuasive parents? Was it running around in the outdoors? skipping? hula hooping? jumping? climbing? dancing? or swimming? The list is endless.

Once you've recalled your childhood passion, then look at ways to incorporate the *essence* of what it was, as much as possible into the activity you choose to take on today.

It might mean taking up a weekly dance class, hiking, an early morning swim, taking up belly dancing classes(the hula hoop connection), or any number of ways to replicate and bring back the joy that once came to you naturally.

Once this is mastered, the sustainability is much greater than a prescription given by someone one who really doesn't know you in your entirety.

There are a variety of activities that do not require you to be at the mercy of a gym membership. I am not negating the benefits of signing up to your local gym facilities, as I too incorporate this into my own regime. However, if you get creative, there are a lot of alternatives to choose from that can give you a multitude of benefits without the additional cost.
What ever you do choose, be mindful of safety first. Where necessary, in the beginning you may benefit from recruiting a hands on guide to show you the ropes.
Thereafter, commit to continue *no matter what.*
Most of all *enjoy* it, make moving something you *look forward to* and you will be amazed at how much you 'lighten up' on many levels.

7. Healing with food first.

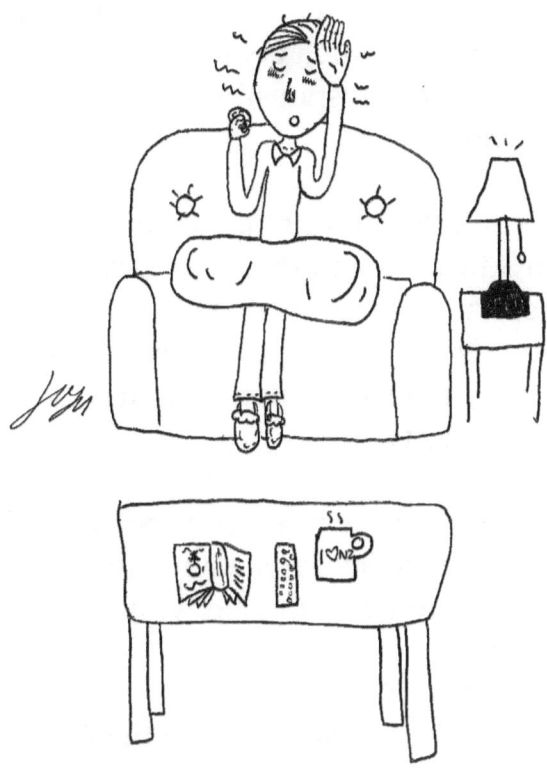

This is a subject which in my opinion, has come a long way over the past decade or so. It does however, still have a long way to go yet before people will readily connect food/drink/lifestyle to their physical manifestations.

In many cultural traditions, nature is the first port of call in order to heal a physical condition, before going the route of prescriptive medication and/or surgery.

I do not negate the great work our overburdened general practitioners, which is performed on a daily basis. They have a profound role in our society and warrant due respect. Unfortunately though, they are generally swamped by trivialities which could be avoided if only people took a little more responsibility for their own personal wellbeing.

Often times, the slightest hint of a cough or a sniffle sends many on a fast track to the pharmacy counter or the waiting room at their local GP's office. Ironically, the waiting room is a prime location for both spreading and picking up any bugs or viruses that may be hankering in its vacinity.

So let's look at a few of the more common complaints people generally seek a Doctor's advice for, and find out how some of them can be addressed with food first.

The common cold:
From as far back as I can remember, in the northern Hemisphere, the dawning of the winter months brought with them coughs, sneezes, runny and crusty noses, squeaky voices and the infamous few days off school due to sleepless nights from being congested. In my family we mistakenly followed the old wives' tale of *'Feed a cold and starve a fever'*. This sentiment wasn't necessarily incorrect, providing the instruction on *what* to feed the cold had been available. What would also have been beneficial is the information on what to *avoid*, in order to speed up the recovery process.
Usually the things that brought the most comfort were really not doing any favours to either our immunity or to

the speed at which we could return to school. ….
perhaps there was an unconscious effort to make the
latter possible!
Here are some simple strategies to address this irritating
and often debilitating occurrence.

Prevention: **Wear appropriate clothing** when seasons
start to change!
I am amazed to see kids going to school in the early
morning winter temperatures, wearing ensembles
likened to what would be suitable for a hot summer
BBQ event. Even the standard school uniform can be
customised to maximise street credit as oppose to being
temperature smart.

Stock up on your body's immunity.
Ensure you are getting plenty of the essential vitamins,
minerals, fresh air, exercise and laughter. Yes, laughter
boosts the body's ability to deal with stress and therefore
helps to boost immunity levels, whatever your age or
gender. And of course hydrate! Plenty of clean fresh
water, often.

Avoid mucus forming Dairy foods & beverages.
Avoiding dairy products whilst having a common cold,
will lessen the common symptoms such as excess mucus
and congestion, as well as reducing inflammatory
conditions that may be accompanied by a stressed
immunity.

Digestive Issues:
Issues with digestion can range from the common
complaint of Heart Burn to Irritable Bowel Syndrome.

If you are dealing with IBS, then I suspect that you have been dealing with this over a period of time and have had it diagnosed from your General Practitioner.

What I will provide here, is information that when applied, can help digestive issues in any stage.

Often times when people eat, they consume a wide range of complex combinations.
The first thing I would suggest is to *simplify*.
Keep the contents of your meal plate as identifiable as possible!

People today are so busy running around attending to everything and everyone, leaving little time to meet their own needs. Then when 'heart burn' or the desire to 'burp' appears, it is often justified with an explanation of being unable to eat offending foods, such as cucumber etc.. Here's what I would encourage in a bid to end the burping trend.

First of all, as I previously mentioned, **simplify**.

Eating a commonly consumed starchy meal combination such as bread, rice, pasta or potatoes, with meat, fish, or other high protein foods, topped with a rich sauce and closely followed by a sugary dessert of any kind, washed down with any variety of beverage, is the digestive equivalent of a high speed train crash. This digestive bombardment, though rather extreme in this instance, is exactly why you might be experiencing indigestion symptoms of varying degrees.

Instead of taking the 'perceived culprit' such as cucumber, onions, garlic or any other commonly accused digestive perpetrators, out of your diet, it would be wise to just make eating a simple, yet nutritious exercise.

Digestive reflux (heart burn) can be linked to not listening to the signal your body gives when you've had enough, eating too fast, drinking with food *(which inhibits the digestive juices from doing the job they are meant to do)*, and of course rushing around whilst 'inhaling' breakfast/lunch in one bite!
I will cover 'conscious eating' a little more later on in the book.

Digestion itself is both a complex and incredibly intelligent process when given the opportunity to do so optimally.
Give your digestive system the best opportunity possible, by being mindful of how quickly, how much, and with what, you ingest in any one meal sitting. In return, it will reward you with a level of health and energy you only ever dreamed of having.

The following are some very beneficial, **natural digestive aids** which come in the form of what regularly grows in the garden, what you can pick up from your local farmers' market, or are readily available in your local food store:

Cumin; - A regularly used spice in various savoury dishes such as stir fry, broths, rice dishes and is also delicious when added to herbal teas with a spoonful of honey.

Peppermint; - Growing, very often uncontrollably, in the garden. This is a delicious addition to any salads, boiled new potatoes, deserts and of course to make tea with. Just add several leaves to boiling water, add a little honey and you've got yourself a quality and nutritious beverage; - Leave it to cool in the fridge for a refreshing drink on a hot summer afternoon.

Peppermint also has the great added benefit of promoting alertness, so a nice one to sip on while in the office or when you're just about to embark on a heady task.

Ginger; - A personal favourite of mine. A warming spice added to several savoury dishes such as curries, samosas, rice dishes and asian cooking.

It is so versatile as it is also used in several sweet dishes and cakes/cookies and scones.

Again, one of the most beneficial ways of getting ginger into your diet is to make tea from it. The most efficient way to extract the flavour from raw root ginger, is to grate the ginger(about the size of a small dice worth, after peeling) into a cup of boiling water, add honey for taste and sip with delight!

Ginger really aids digestion and as an added bonus, helps mobilise fat, therefore can assist as part of a healthy weight loss regime.

Be aware though, ginger has diuretic properties and can therefore mean that when drinking this fine beverage close to bed time, slightly interrupted sleep may ensue, due to having to get up for a bathroom visit or two!

Also, because of it's diuretic properties, you will need to make sure your are properly hydrated to compensate.

Additional tip for digestive aid:

One of the most soothing practices, which I personally use regularly, is to apply a soothing 'clockwise direction' massage to your abdomen. This can be done with any natural oil, though my preference leans towards either coconut oil or sesame oil(not toasted). This creates a flow for the digestive system and can stimulate relief from a whole range of symptoms, from constipation, premenstrual cramps, tension cramps due to stress, bloating and gas. The best time to do this is first thing in the morning.

Blood sugar issues:
Some examples of issues relating to blood sugar, range from frequent low blood sugar, blood sugar fluctuations/ energy dips, to diabetes and metabolic syndrome.
This is an area where it pays to take a good look at the bigger picture. In order to get your blood sugar levels under control, it is vital to maintain a consistently stable and nutritious eating plan.
Very often when experiencing an energy 'dip', the tendency is to reach for a 'quick fix'. This regularly comes in the form of something sugary, white flour baked products(eg biscuits, cakes and baked food items), coffee or a sugary drink.
What follows is an energy 'boost' which is very short lived. It is not only short lived, it retreats to beyond what the original level of energy was when you first reached for the 'solution'. And so the cycle begins, in a never ending yo yo of peaks and troughs.
Cycles like these lead to constant trips to the food cupboard, refrigerator or local grocery store, creating

havoc with insulin production and can, over time, lead to the dreaded diabetes.

Diabetes is sneaking its way through generations and is now beginning to show up all too often in the younger school-going age groups. This needs to be addressed now, while there is still time.
Some ideas for blood sugar solutions;

Cinnamon; Added to virtually *anything* and *everything*, will provide sweetness and a warm comforting flavour, while stabilising blood sugar - avoiding the 'spike' in insulin in the process.

Snack on high protein foods; Instead of reaching for a quick fix 'health bar'(remember the 'health bar' I mentioned earlier?), try snacking on something with a higher protein content, such as nuts, seeds or a little cube of quality cheese.

Headaches and Migraine:
This is a pretty complex subject and has equally as many complex explanations for the causes and degree of symptoms. For anyone who suffers from either regular headaches or the occasional (or frequent) migraine, then there are some basic ways to tackle and alleviate this debilitating and unnecessary common challenge.

For many of our common day to day ailments, there is a food to reach for which will in some way help to alleviate the condition. When it comes to headaches/

migraines however, it is what you can *take out* of your diet that can result in a noticeable positive outcome.

As we all know, stress is one of the biggest challenges as a result of the pace of life today. This will often manifest, in this instance, as a headache/migraine.

So, the first stop shop is to recognise *what* is causing stress to this degree.

Tackle it head on (pun intended), deal with the stressful situation and get it over with. Headaches can also show up when there are little nagging remnants of either anger, resentment, fear or guilt, which you may not even be consciously aware of.

So, dig deep and find out what it's really about and again, deal with it, diffuse it, release it, let it go, forgive it and move on!

Of course, one of the best ways to alleviate stress is to get your body moving, in whatever way you feel like you can. Dance, run, walk, swim, skip, race up a flight of stairs, get the vacuum cleaner out and cover two challenges in one go!

Note; To date, unfortunately cleaning has not yet made the category of a sport form, however, it has all the benefits similar to that of attending a low impact aerobics class, without having to leave the house!

You may also opt for the gentler approach and treat yourself to a de stressing massage or equivalent.

Some really beneficial things to include on a regular basis to balance the ill-effect of stress are;

Foods high in Vitamin B

Some of the more common sources are; whole grains, nuts, seeds, seafood, pumpkin, greens, eggs, meat(if you are a meat eater, otherwise get creative with increasing vegetable and legumes(beans) consumption), yeast products, avocados, broccoli & asparagus, to name a few. Calming foods & herbs such as; sage, lemon balm, chamomile, and the 'wonder spice' turmeric.

Food related items to eliminate in order to address the issue of Headaches and/or Migraines;

The obvious one would of course be **Caffeine.** I am not suggesting that caffeine has a similar effect on every individual. It is rather, something to be treated with respect and reverence. It is a case of *a little* is a wonderful accompaniment to an enjoyable conversation with friends, and too much can contribute to becoming tired but wired.

Start to recognising how *sensitive* your own body is to caffeine, then adjust intake accordingly, until ideally, it is eliminated.

Sugar is another item to avoid and/or eliminate when experiencing headaches/migraines. Actually, this is one to permanently wipe out of your existence and here's why.

Sugar's addictive properties (and it has been likened to that of addiction to cocaine), together with its inviting taste, has most of us hooked. *Eating even a small amount creates the desire for more.*

If you just take a look at the ingredient list on most of the average packaged foods in the majority of households, sugar shows up in various forms. It is masqueraded as sucrose, glucose, invert sugar, corn syrup, fructose, pectin, and the list goes on, mostly combined with that which we cannot either pronounce or understand the effects of.

Harsh as it sounds, when it comes to this toxic white substance, being harsh is absolutely necessary. Especially if you are to free yourself from the lure of the sweet stuff permanently.

Sugar can be incredibly toxic, and when consumed in frequent and large quantities, it will have longterm detrimental effects on your health. There is no 'sugar coated' method of getting this message across.

So where does this message fit into alleviating headaches?

One of the side effects of the sugar load is headaches. Simple. So reduce and even better, get rid of it!

As a rule of thumb, anything reading over 6g of sugar on an ingredient list, should be questioned. Will the instant gratification of taste and energy spike, be worth the after effects of the deep energy lull and the need for more?

Note; for each 4g of sugar listed on the 'per serve' nutritional information label, it is equal to 1 whole teaspoonful of sugar.

This information is no doubt familiar to some, as there are copious resources to reiterate the message of the need to let go of sugar. So for now, let's just see this as a little guidance to help you free your mind and 'lighten' your body!

Something that often goes unnoticed is *how* food ends up the way it does, in the supermarket shelves, in those shiny brightly coloured packages, cans and boxes. I am no scientist, but I have come to the conclusion that if food didn't have some kind of 'chemical interference' from when it first appeared in nature, to the 'altered' state in which it shows up in the supermarket, then we would be looking at some seriously rotting produce on the shelves.

It is not surprising therefore, that your body often protests when it's bombarded with items it cannot recognise as 'real food' and doesn't have the equipment to do anything other than file it under the 'toxin' category, only to show up later in the form of cellulite, mood swings, skin issues, and of course **headaches**.

Colouring & Preservatives;

Some people admittedly are a little less sensitive than others to the many combinations of substances used to preserve and colour the food we see on the shelves today. However, that doesn't make it any less detrimental to the health of those individuals. It may show up for them at a later stage, as excess weight, grumpiness and with the addition of addictive tendencies.

Many experience headaches/migraines at the mere taste of some of the culprits (such as MSG for example). So here is my straight forward guide when it comes to getting chemicals out of your diet and back in science labs where they belong.

If you don't understand an ingredient or can't pronounce it, don't buy it!

If it is so brightly and perfectly coloured that it begs admiration, and is *not* a fresh fruit or vegetable item, steer clear!

Again, a little harsh, but I endeavour to help you alleviate common complaint that is the frequent headache.

Chemical cocktails; are found not only amongst various food items, but throughout the home. A combination of the following can, *over time*, create a toxic environment that can invite symptoms such as **headaches, migraines,** allergies, and asthma.

Items such as:
Cleaning chemicals, Air fresheners (yes, even those lovely scented candles!), Gas fires (when overused), and if I were to get really picky, too much time spent around computers, mobile phones and wireless technology.
Another place to look out for chemical culprits is in your personal care products. Aerosol sprays, perfumes, make up, shower products and body lotions.

I'm not suggesting that you start clearing out your home right now and stop personal hygiene. What I *am* suggesting is that you start looking at ways to reduce the implications of a build up of and combination of the examples mentioned.

Pain:
Pain is the body's final message to you, letting you know that something needs attention. It is a signal that somewhere in your body there is *inflammation.* Very often though, by the time it shows up as pain, the common trend is to rush for either pain killers or line up in the Doctor's waiting room.
As for any physical ailment or issue, prevention is always best.

What has become very apparent today, is the multitude of 'inflammatory promoting' foods that are consumed on a regular basis.

Surprisingly, they are very often the things which are viewed as 'pretty healthy', but when consumed *regularly* and *over time,* contribute to the multitude of inflammatory eventualities such as;   Obesity, Heart disease, Diabetes, Cancer, Alzheimer's and Stroke, to name a few.

The foods in question are those that are highly processed. Unfortunately, as too are the common 'hot of the bakery shelf' foods. Couple this with an over consumption of starchy foods, especially the white starches like potatoes, breads, pastas and rice, and it is a recipe for an inflammatory process. That isn't to say that they may never appear on your plate again, it is the *regularity* and *quantity* consumed that makes a difference.

So again, finding a *balance* in *what*, *how often* and *how much*, is really the way forward in order to avoid deprivation or obsession.

The best way to deal with and **prevent inflammation** is to make ensure you have an adequate regular intake of *high quality* omega 3 giving foods.   Some examples of such are; fish oil, wild salmon, sardines, walnuts, avocado, anchovies, flaxseed.

Other examples of anti-inflammatory foods are ;-
Kelp / Turmeric(in my opinion a 'wonder' spice) / Shiitake mushrooms / Green Tea (let's not forget though that green tea does contain a little caffeine as well as it's health giving properties) / Papaya / Blueberries (who'd

have thought it!) / extra virgin Olive Oil / Broccoli /
Sweet Potato.

As well as including a healthy proportion of all of these
recommended foods, the commonly recognised 'health
promoter', is of course, exercise; done *moderately* and
consistently, when combined with a balanced approach
to addressing stress, the need to partake in the
contribution to our General Practitioner's workload is
greatly reduced.

8. Conscious Eating.

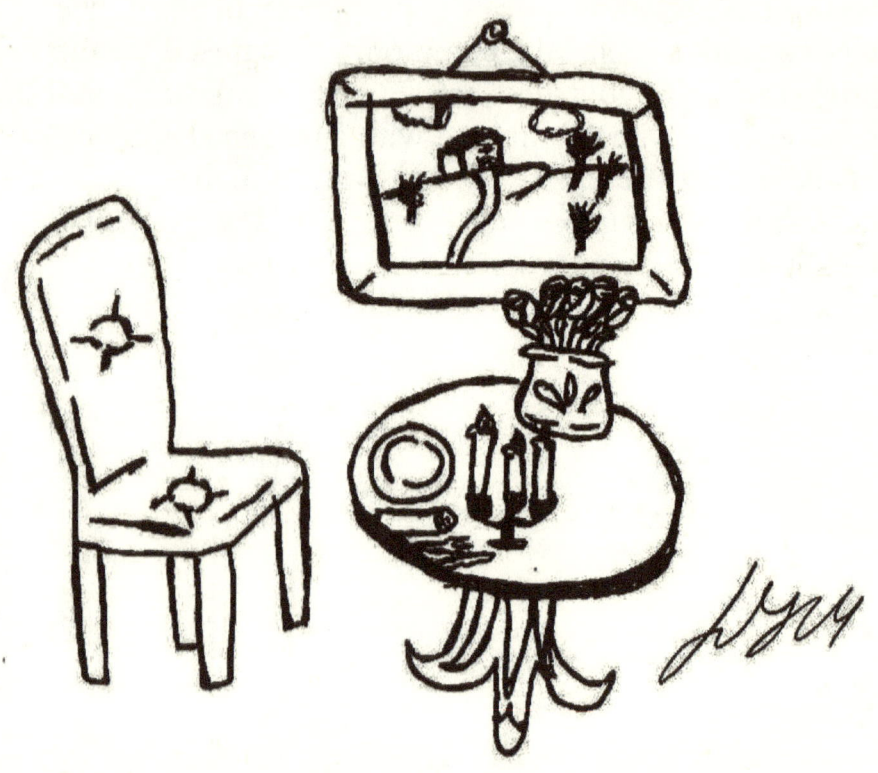

It could be questioned 'how could I possibly eat if I were unconscious?', which in its literal sense is a fair question. What I am going to discuss here, is the state of 'mindlessness' or 'not really paying attention' when eating.

At a guess, I would confidently say that we are all either guilty of 'unconscious eating', have been known to partake in, or will definitely slip into, minutes of unconscious eating at some stage of our lives.

I have always loved food, since as far back as I can remember. I loved the sight, smell and most of all, the taste. It would be fair to say that I formed a 'relationship' with food from a very early age. I viewed it as both a yummy experience to settle hunger, or as a comforting escape... (escape from the noise and often raucous environment that accompanied living with 4 sisters, 2 brothers, Mum, Dad, *Great Auntie Maggie, a collection of dairy farm animals which included cows, pigs, chickens, turkeys, and a border collie..).

Often my meals took on the heat of a personal race against time, before my scrounging brothers spotted what was not yet eaten on my plate and assumed it was perfectly acceptable to reach across and swipe the last piece of fatty bacon or equivalent right off my plate. As far as I was concerned, eating became a mission of being able to eat fast enough so that I could retain my portion of the daily fare.

The emotional roller coaster began way before actually sitting down to the overcrowded rectangular formica 'foldable' table, which housed enough comfortable chairs for the 'older' siblings, often leaving the unstable tiny foldable chair for the 'baby'! Indeed, being the youngest sibling, I was always addressed as 'the baby'. Unaware then, that it is perfectly acceptable for a child to express the inner turmoil and question his or her contribution and value within the pack, I remained silent

*and 'watchful' in the hope that I would not be placed
next to either brother.*

*I also mistakenly formed the conclusion very early on,
that 'feeding men' took priority. This conclusion came
from the evidence I collected in my silent observation of
the countless times our farm was being tended to by a
hand picked select few 'great farm workers' that my Dad
held trustworthy enough to help around harvesting &/or
hay time. Those were jobs that he took so much pride in
and wrapped his existence around.*
*I deeply dreaded those periods of what felt like
'intrusion' in our household, not only because I could
sense that they were impinging on the structure I had
come to depend on, but because Mum always insisted on
'feeding the men first'!*

*Given this principal, it could easily have been
somewhere deep in the Indian Hinterland! But like
religion, adult conversations including money, sex,
contraception and the importance of not letting anyone
know what you really feel, this was not questioned.*
*As I watched the last succulent sausage slide delicately
off the frying pan, a waft of onions cooked in bacon fat
ready for the addition of mashed turnip, parsnip or
carrots, I held back the sting of a tear, knowing that we
would end up with a quick 'makeshift' version of the
piping hot fresh mound of potatoes, veggies, bacon &/or
sausages.*
*As I glared through tear-stained eyes, at the unfairness
of their misguided gender importance, I could already
feel the knots beginning in my empty tummy. When it
was finally my turn to eat, I doubt if I could even taste*

what had made its way onto my plate. I shovelled with a frenzy of anger. Anger that I had to wait, anger that I had not been made equal and anger that it was not as hot as I wanted it to be.

That's enough trauma to create a life long series of digestive issues, complicated relationships with food and a host of issues relating to the complimentary sex! All of which I have, in turn, touched upon to a lesser or more degree throughout my life.

However, even though my recollection leans towards a kind of rain cloud, there were by contrast, equally as many happy, connected and family bonding moments (without all the 'huggey' bits, as we were never much of a tactile family).

*Some years later, I also remember how I would 'flush with embarrassment' if I bumped into anyone when I was 'on the run, bite in mouth and the rest in hand'! The epitome of mindless and unconscious eating. But several years on, after a lot of soul searching, self-healing, a little counselling and a touch of therapy, I resolve to the fact now that, it really **is** better to sit down before embarking on anything of the nourishing nature.*

Not only is it not a good look, to be running around with remnants of food hanging from your mouth, it really is better for your body when actual time is taken to pay attention to what, where, and how much you are eating.

The common thread that joins these examples right from the outset, is a *lack of consciousness* around what is innately one of the most nourishing acts you can do for yourself.

Here are just a few of the ways that unconsciousness when eating might creep into your life;

Do not assume that I have become enlightened and no longer encounter moments of 'unconscious munching', as like you, I am human and a work in progress.

However, I do lean more towards nourishment than frequent episodes of instant gratification.

Examples of unconscious eating;

Eating while watching TV.   Eating while driving. Eating while talking on the phone (not nice for the person who has to listen to muffled crunching, slopping or chewing!). Eating while working on the computer or just browsing the internet.   Eating when not really hungry. Eating after the hunger has been satisfied. Eating standing up or walking around.

Nibbling when cooking (same as eating when standing up but seemingly more acceptable). Eating that which we know will harm our bodies. Eating an excess of any one food (unless it's kale! however if there is a distorted relationship making you just focus on this one food, then this too slots into 'unconsciousness'). Eating for the 'journey' - car/train/airplane/bus - *This was a personal favourite in the past. I could easily consume an entire packet of rice cakes (yes, without topping - what was I thinking!) on the twenty minute train ride home from work. On these occasions I would leave the station with a slightly spacey and irritable energy. If you are unfamiliar with the feeling accompanied by an overload of simple carbohydrates, then this would be a good representation.*

So how can 'unconscious eating' also contribute to being overweight?

Lots of factors are at play here.

Firstly, if the speed at which you are eating is consistently high, you won't have sufficient time between the food entering your mouth and entering your stomach, to register that you have had enough. It takes 10-15 minutes for this procedure to take place and whilst you are 'tuning out' the signal pathway, you have no true indication of when enough is enough. In which case, you unknowingly continue to 'fill up'.

How many times have you heard, or said "I'm full now" or "I Couldn't eat another bite? Unfortunately when this stage has been reached, it's already too late. You have filled up *more* than to full capacity. This is the result of the last bite going in as the stomach was already trying to give the satiety signal, and now there's even more on the way!

A smart guideline to follow, though often difficult, is to practice *slowing down* and *chewing*. Slowing down helps your digestion have a better chance of doing it's job optimally. Plus, you are likely to eat less quantity as a result.

By *chewing your food until it is liquid* before swallowing, there is less likelihood of whole undigested food particles to escape down the digestive track, causing bloating, gas, pain, indigestion or worse case scenario, leaky gut syndrome.

If there is emotional tension, stress or conflict at the time of eating, this puts your digestive system on shut down in a bid to reserve energy for the perceived 'conflict' at hand. This results in an increased *fat storage* as oppose to metabolising food for energy whilst *burning* fat. Have you ever eaten a meal cooked by someone who was in a 'strop', who was angry, moody, throwing utensils around in a 'Gordon Ramsey' frenzy? (ok, so we're all guilty of *some* of those occasionally......); but think about what happens when this sort of energy is transferred into our precious bodies. It may sound a little far fetched to some of you, and that's perfectly ok, but many will recognise the necessity to pursue 'peace in the kitchen' and 'peace at the dining table'.

Remember also, the digestion's *intention* is to efficiently process food in an orderly manner. If you are stressed, the body's response switches to hang onto food as fat in case of an emergency, as in that moment it doesn't feel safe to perform the important task of optimal digestion. Can you see how this, *over time* and done *consistently*, affects the waistline?

When I think of 'conscious eating', I often bring to mind my dear Great Auntie Maggie, who we were fortunate enough be able to share our home with for her last fifteen years before she passed away. She was the epitome of elegance, confidence and pure grace itself. What often mesmerised me, was when I watched her perform her little 'milk and bread' routine. Her 'before bedtime' snack was hot milk, a little cinnamon, a small piece of freshly baked white bread coated in sugar. What? White bread? sugar? Indeed. I believe that the

fact that she was so elegantly slender, was the result of
*her **consciousness** with **how** she ate.*

The milk was poured into a delicate china cup which
was placed on a saucer. The bread cut into tiny strips
like wafers, the sugar dusted lightly on top and the
cinnamon subtly creating the aroma of pure goodness.
(this probably explains my love of cinnamon today). As
she dipped the bread into the milk (Not so elegant I hear
you say. But she could be forgiven due to her extended
little finger!). She delicately ate in tiny bites, chewing,
chewing, chewing, until her body decided that she had
enough. When asked the question of whether she had
had enough, her frequent response was, "That was
superfluous, any more and it would be flittery flattery"..
This still makes me smile today, as well as providing a
gentle reminder to *slow down* and *listen* to when I have
had enough, regardless of how delicious it tastes or how
much is left over.

So, *how* you eat plays just as important a role as *what*
you eat.

Here are a few little tasks to get you on your way to
becoming a 'mindful eater'.

1. Before putting a morsel into your mouth, stop and
    check if you are indeed hungry. Check where you
    are on a hunger scale of 1 to 10 (1 being totally full
    and 10 being that your tummy is empty and
    grumbling). If you registered between 1 and 5, I
    suspect that you are craving for something that no
    amount of food will satisfy. If this is so, it could be
    time to head out for a walk, phone a friend, de-clutter
    a drawer or cupboard, hug your children &/your

partner and my favourite strategy is to drink a large glass of water. Often times you could just be de-hydrated, which can confusingly show up masquerading as hunger. If you registered between 6 and 10, then you do indeed need to eat.

2. Now that you have established that you are going to eat something, it is time to select/prepare/order/ or unwrap your chosen nourishment. Select according to two criteria. Firstly, that it is something you genuinely *like* the taste of, and secondly, that it is as nutritious and health giving as possible. After all, this choice will determine how you will feel physically and emotionally, approximately twenty minutes to an hour after eating it.

3. Sit down!! The car does not count unless you have actually stopped the car, taken off your seatbelt, assumed a stress free posture and have no distractions in sight.

4. Take a moment to look at your food. Take a moment to smell your food. Take a moment to take a deep breath and if even if you are not religious, take a moment to acknowledge and give thanks for what you are about to eat. If that sounds a little too 'zen' or ambitious for a large family clambering to get to the table, then it can be done very subtly and very 'silently' in just a moment's thought.

5. When it's time to start the journey from mouth to stomach, do it without anything else weaving its way into the process, such as background TV sounds, phone, laptop, ipad, book or newspaper. This might be challenging for those who like to savour the Sunday morning newspaper while munching their way through a Sunday fry up, or for those who like to

multitask. *Working*, whether on the computer or sorting through paperwork, is *not* part of this mindful eating exercise, and should be kept separate at all times.

6. Take smaller mouthfuls. A fantastic way to get to grips with taking smaller mouthfuls of food, is to use chopsticks. A skill in itself and a super way to ensure that there is no chance of overloading in the process. A similar outcome can be had from using smaller utensils.

7. Chew, chew, chew and then chew some more! Somewhere at some time or another, you will have heard the sentiment, 'chew your food a hundred times'! Whilst one hundred times may not be the *exact* number proposed, it isn't far off. Chew until the food forms a liquid consistency, then swallow. It is a difficult one to get the hang of at first, simply because people are so familiar with 'bite-chew-swallow-bite-chew(a little)-swallow....' This kind of eating practice can lead to a never ending stream of complaints, such as indigestion, bloating and gas. *Remember, there are no teeth in your stomach*! The importance of this one act cannot be emphasised enough, as the digestion process starts in the mouth. In fact, even before a morsel is placed there, just the sight, smell and anticipation of food awakens the senses to already begin the digestive process. This is where the term of phrase 'My mouth is watering' comes from, as in fact it really *is* watering, in preparation for the food to follow.

8. I you have followed the plan so far, you are already on your way to being more aware of your satiety signal. In terms of health benefits, and resulting

weight stabilisation, stop eating when you are about 80% full. This provides the remaining 20% with enough space in a healthy environment to complete the digestive process efficiently. When food is processed efficiently, it no longer sits in your stomach creating the infamous bloating, heart burn, lethargy, gas or constipation. When this process is 'moving' in the right direction, you will be rewarded with a healthy and efficient body, increased energy and a narrower waistline. Win win!

This 'mindful' presence, can be adopted for any activity you do. It just requires a little practice, a little effort, a desire to be a healthier individual, and a lot of patience with yourself as you drift in and out of 'consciousness' throughout the task in hand.
So try it first with food, then take it to the Laundry! or the dishes! or wherever else you do routinely on 'auto pilot'.

9. Quality vs Quantity.

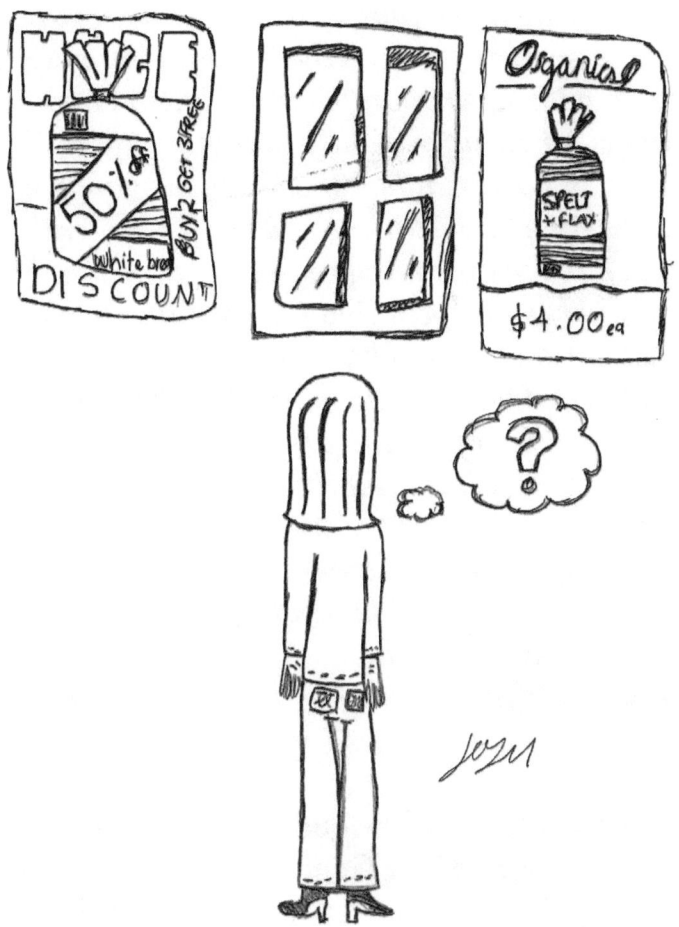

I remember back in the late 70s, when I was just starting out in the world and fending for myself. I had a friend who pretty much took me under her wing, pointing me in the right direction now and again, especially in the areas where I was a little naive.

To my horror, she would regularly spend hundreds of pounds sterling on items such as handbags, shoes or accessories. Back then one hundred pounds sterling was considered an expensive purchase. However, I would happily wade my way through the bargain basements and come up with several outfits including a couple of pairs of boots for as little as fifty pounds or less. Whilst I would gasp in horror at her sheer extravagance and lack of knowledge about where to shop, she relentlessly tried to teach me the meaning of quality over quantity. For her, there was no substitute for spending hard earned cash on something that was going to go the distance. I guess I was a little more short sighted and wanted regular instant gratification at the expense of things falling apart all too soon.

Slowly but surely as the years progressed, I look back at those days with pure admiration and gratitude for the lessons learnt, and whilst I haven't become a 'designer' girl with a 'passion for fashion,' I have very much embraced the enjoyment and satisfaction of choosing quality in many of the choices I make today.

What has this got to do with food? As the very talented Author, Teacher & Speaker Geneen Roth says, **"The way we do *anything* is the way we do *everything*"**.

When it comes down to it, the foods you feed yourself and the beverages you drink, are no different from the things you embrace daily. Things such as relationships, home environment, social interaction and lifestyle choices.

There have been many changes throughout the last few decades in relation to the quality of the food available and the extensive range of *fake*, *processed* and *genetically altered* items that now line the shelves of our supermarkets. Not only is this creating confusion about what you are actually eating, it also drives the emotional charge to reach for convenience *and* perhaps what is on special offer from moment to moment.

For many, the dollar will be the deciding factor in what goes into the fridge and cupboards for any given week. I would however, encourage even the most thrifty of shoppers, to pause for a moment and take stock of *why* in fact some of these products are on 'special' and *whom* they are targeting.

I have already touched on this topic early on in 'Navigating the Supermarket'.   However, it is worth revisiting for the purpose of driving home the message and giving you back your personal power for your weekly grocery shopping.

Most of the 'special offer' items, especially those which target young children, have little or no nutritional value whatsoever. I would even go as far as to say that many of them contain a cocktail of ingredients manipulated for the prime purpose of wanting kids to keep coming back for more.

So the *nutritional quality* in many items that are targeted to children, with their brightly coloured packaging and their promise of fun and laughter, is often at the expense of *quantity* and for example, how many packs you can buy for under $5!

Let's re-explore the concept of eating organically. Many people shy away from this concept due to the seemingly unbalanced economical bottom line, opting instead for the supermarket and corner shop alternatives.

The following are a couple of suggestions which I encourage you to experiment with, that may help you to gradually shift to better quality choices:

1. If you are currently predominantly buying non-organic fresh produce from the supermarket, start swapping one item per month for the organic version. You will notice of course, that there is a price difference. So with this in mind, look at combining the chosen vegetable with other non-organic vegetables, but use *less* than you do currently. (If you *are* buying non-organic fruits and vegetables, one way to help lessen the detrimental effects of chemical pesticide sprays is to soak the fruits/vegetables in water with added vinegar and a little baking soda. Then rinse thoroughly before cooking/eating).

2. You can adapt the 'progressive swapping' concept to any additional non-organic produce, such as eggs, dairy, meats, etc. Consider if you are regularly having non-organic meat 3-4 times per week, switching to a *good quality organic meat* and have this just *once* per week. You will not only improve your health in the long term, but it will significantly reward you financially.

When looking at the quantity of food *necessary* to feed an average individual, it is surprisingly lower than what is currently being consumed. Much of this can be linked to the mass production of branded food items and the new availability of any food at any time of year due to it's intense processing and storage ability.

An abundance of food has very quickly transferred onto the plates of the nations, and subsequently surrounds the internal organs of a large percentage of the population, giving expansion to the 'once narrow' waistlines.

Habits are very easily incorporated into every day life and unless conscious effort is put into changing these, they become part of who we are and what we have become.

The oversized dinner plates and portion sizes that are now regularly gracing the plates of the majority of households, are no longer reserved for special occasions. I say this with the utmost empathy and understanding, as someone who has also experienced portion size increasing over the years.

*On reflection, even as a child I had the ability to consume a vast amount of food. So much so that Mum would often comment on the possibility that I might have worms!(I didn't), or would sometimes ask, "where does it all go?" or "are you **still** eating?"......*
Not the most positive and nourishing comments to receive, as an already vulnerable and sensitive young girl struggling to fit into the world in it's complexities.

I have had the honour of listening to some of the most influential teachers and speakers throughout my journey to balanced health. They have all expressed the common sentiment that we should *systematically under eat* in order to remain healthy and live a quality, long and fulfilling life.

For many this will wave a red flag of 'deprivation' or 'instruction to become anorexic or obsessively thin'. So let me quickly assure you that it is solely a recommendation for people to eat just *a little less* than they are doing now, *on a consistent basis,* until you are eating like goldilocks "not too much, not too little, just enough!"

10. Stop Comparing...*there only is one you!*

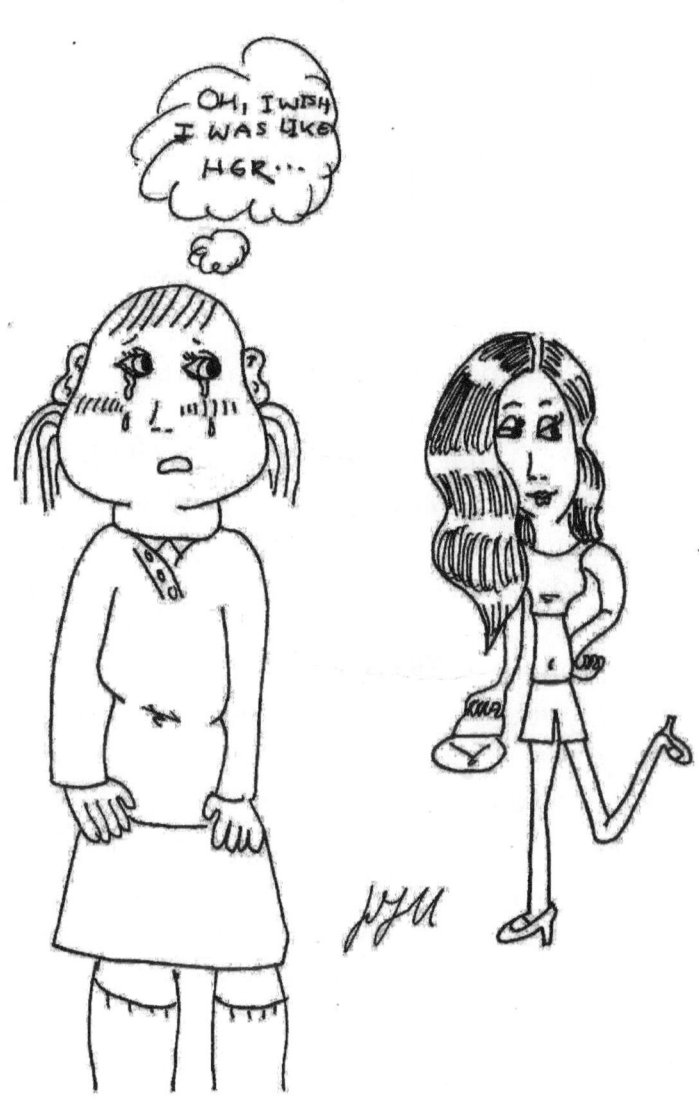

For those of you like myself, who are one of several siblings, you will no doubt at some point in your upbringing, have experienced the heart-sinking mutterings of comparison. The most heart-sinking of all, is that from your parents themselves, topped only by the often snide and hurtful power play of *siblings,* whose seeming apparent role in life is to make you wish you had never been born.

If however, you are an only child, so long as there are individuals of a similar age and gender in the world, then you are not exempt from the pangs of self doubt and inner criticism.

It starts from the moment you notice the admiring eyes of your entrusted parent or caregiver towards another individual, and from that moment the belief that 'I need to be more, or be like *them* in order to be loved' starts to show up in various forms, for as long as you allow it to. It probably sounds like I have been a candidate for a lifetime of therapy! Admittedly, there have been times during my stumbles through adolescence and early adulthood that I would have agreed, and to be honest, a lot of my inner processing and healing has come from my own investigation, trials and errors.
I have also roamed from teacher to teacher, healer to healer, guru to guru, only to eventually realise that I *already* have and *always have had*, what is necessary in order to be the person I am today.
The me who is unique, sometimes a bit batty, a little neurotic at times, sometimes catching myself being a control freak, but at the end of the day, that's what

makes me who I am and no one else is ever going to be Colette.

Everyone has a purpose for their unique individuality. Including the foods that suit your individual body, and the thoughts you furnish your mind with both consciously and unconsciously. You have *your own* path to take which can be a huge responsibility, but you get to make the choices in every thing you do, everything you eat, everything you drink and everything you think.

You may be familiar with the Victor Frankel imprisonment story and how he did not allow the torture he endured to colour his *response* to the situation. Only *he* had the responsibility to do this.

So what does this have to do with comparing yourself to the images that are splattered across every media stream in today's obsessive and material world? The message is simple, it is not what you see, hear or read about that drives what you do. It is the message you *interoperate* from it which dictates the direction of self acceptance and appreciation, or self-criticism & self-destruct.

But let's face it, it's not that easy is it? Especially so when participating in your regular zumba, step class or equivalent, where you are regularly reminded that size *zero* really *has* crept into every corner of your existence, with the exception of your own wardrobe!
Not only that, but do they also need to rush into class finishing off some rather unhealthy half-eaten giant chocolate-chip cookie? Especially as you have had to muster up every ounce of will power in order to pass by

even the 'healthy cereal bar' section of the grocery store, on your way to class, clutching your 'calorie free, fat free, bottle of yummy water'!

Incidentally, the thing to bear in mind here is that no matter what size is printed on the label of the perfectly fitting hipsters, *eating on the run* or eating *heavily processed and high sugar laden snacks*, will come back to bite hard! Perhaps not immediately, but *over time* certainly. (review previous chapter on conscious eating). Back to your class...

The conversation which ensues in that moment of passive confrontation, is more often than not likened to some of the following examples;

"I want to be like that' "I want to be able to show up at class having shovelled down a few hundred calories and not have to worry about being two sizes bigger by the time class ends" "I wish I didn't have to wear a baggy t'shirt to cover up my muffin top or my monthly bulge".

Take a moment right now and stop! Take a deep breath, now take another. For just a moment, bring all your attention to what is going on in *your* body. Can you recall how many times you felt that you were 'less than', that you were 'too this' 'too that', 'not good enough', 'not slim enough'?

If there is any kind of tension or tightness anywhere, around the shoulders, in your tummy, in your legs, your arms & hands; just *let it go*...take another big deep nourishing breath in, filling up with clean fresh and nourishing oxygen, then exhale all the tension, non-nourishing thoughts and feelings.

Let it go.

Ok, so I sneaked in that little process just to provide you with a handy little tool that you can take with you anywhere. Any time you recognise those thoughts of comparison creep in, stop, in the moment, and breathe.

Feelings and habitual thoughts of comparison like those mentioned, don't just appear over night. You didn't suddenly wake up and go from loving and accepting yourself unconditionally, to feeling like you are bottom of the pack.

So are they likely to go away over night? No. The sooner you can start to question those thoughts and *beliefs* about yourself and whether they are nourishing you or punishing you, the sooner you will have found the turning point on the yellow brick road of self acceptance, and self love.

Given that the complete turnaround is not going to happen instantaneously, what can you start doing to move in the direction of self accepting bliss?

Firstly, take a long hard, objective and *uncritical* look at what *is*. Ask the question 'What are the things I *cannot* change, no matter what? The answer to this question varies according to how extensive your desire to go under the knife is, given that in today's world, someone somewhere can, no doubt, alter *anything* you desire!.... But at what price? Let me be clear here, I am not condoning going down this route. It is a choice that begs extensive investigation and even then, there are never any guarantees!......I digress..

Some examples of features you *absolutely cannot change,* are;

If you are 5'2" tall you will *never* be 6ft. Additional things that will never change are your bone structure and unique body shape. Body shape, through diet & lifestyle changes, is something which can be *enhanced*, but your individual bone structure and underlying shape will *not* change.

Accepting this, can be one of the most liberating gifts you can give yourself. No longer will you wile away the hours of frustrating and pointless attempts to emulate the unattainable media portrayals of 'perfection'.

Let's look now at some of the things you *can* do something about.
It will require *taking action*!!!!
How many times have you complained about how your skin is dull, your hair is frizzy or dry, your nails are brittle, or most commonly, you need help zipping up your favourite summer shorts!
The good news is you can change *all* of these! If you have been digesting what you have read so far, you will already have started to experience little changes.
You may no longer crave that sugar binge at 3pm in the afternoon. You may no longer have to wade your way through packets of processed paraphernalia to get to the *real* food in your pantry, or you may be already reconnecting with your long lost skinny pants which you retrieved from the back of your closet!

If so, well done! fantastic job! If not? no problem. In the words of Eckhart Tolle…"*The point of power is always now*".

Let's not waste any more time or energy with 'should have' or 'if only'. Just commit to beginning *now.*
Begin by choosing the things that you *most* want to change. The things that you *do* have control of and *can* physically do something about. Then get it underway!

You will want the changes you are about to create to be sustainable and with you for the long haul, so don't try to do everything at once. Commit to taking small steps *consistently,* then *over time,* the rewards will greet you in abundance.
Be excited. Your amazing journey has already begun, so enjoy the ride.

11. Suggested Recipes.

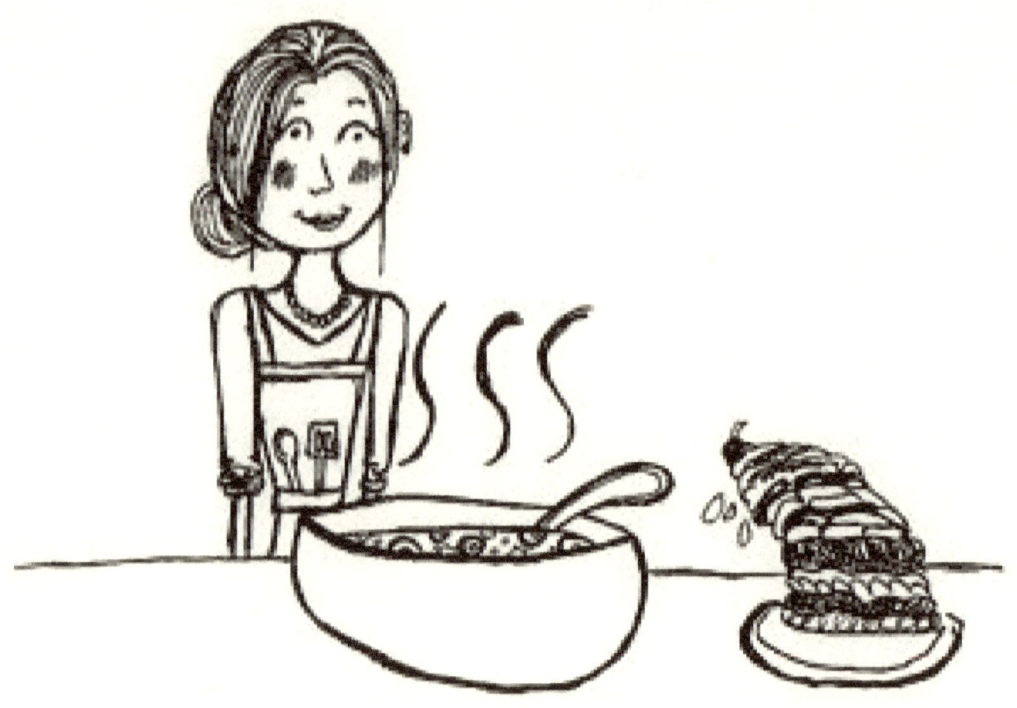

I stalled for a moment when it came to this chapter, simply because I wanted to find a way of providing recipes, without *strict instructions* to be followed to the letter, labelling them *Colette's* Recipes. Instead, I would prefer if you were able to create something that you could call your own. Something that you can 'tweak' here and there according to what mood you are in, what your flavour preferences are on the day, and according to what foods are in your pantry at the time.

So I came up with a plan. I will walk you through some of the popular dishes I put together for myself, my husband and our 14yr old daughter. They are largely experimentation each day I make them and my family have grown to rather love my little creations, including the many dishes that do not yet have a name.
As I write the ingredients and methods, I will also give some indications of where you can make the dish your own.

The last thing you need when time is of the essence, is to be opening a glossy recipe book and following the steps necessary to make a dish that would win awards on Top Chef, but has taken 3 hours to prepare!

I am all for spending your time wisely, putting as much energy into a *condensed* amount of focused activity, leaving space and time to fill with the simple pleasures life presents, but that you are often too busy to notice.

A forewarning though, when it comes to combinations on Toast or Rice Cakes, I can be a little eccentric, or as my daughter would refer to it as being "*just weird*"! Sometimes I just can't decide what to put on my toast, or rice cake. I might have so many tastes that I want to experience that I need to spread them all. I often allocate 'little compartments' so that I can cater for the many tastes I hanker after at the time.
This, understandably is not to everyone's taste, however, I encourage you to experiment with simple things that

you wouldn't have dreamed of putting together, or thought that they were only to be combined if you are a 6 year old.

I recollect a time back in the UK in my early twenties, when I lived amongst what I can only describe as a kind of 'creatively starved' and 'extremely conservative' family. Like clockwork, each Sunday was celebrated with the traditional Sunday Lunch. This consisted of the infamous 'roast', accompanied by roast potatoes, vegetables, gravy and the star of the Sunday show, the Yorkshire pudding. For those who are unfamiliar with Yorkshire Pudding, it is a northern UK delicacy made from batter, baked in a muffin tray containing piping hot fat, the hotter the better (obviously oblivious to the dangers of trans fats back then), and served with the Sunday roast. Traditionally the gravy would be strategically poured into the 'valley-like' centre of the pudding.

Even back then, my creative taste buds came out to play and on one occasion I asked if I could have my Yorkshire Pudding with syrup and ice cream? An unforgivable mistake on my part! My request was firmly rejected and referred to as 'sacrilege'.

Let's begin with what I would refer to as the most important meal of the day;

Breakfast.

The word in itself indicates the *break*ing of *fast*, unless of course you've spent the night sleepwalking into the kitchen and indulging from the pantry and/or the fridge.

Breakfast is personally my favourite meal. I even admit to having on occasions, gone to bed filled with excitement at the thought of what next morning's fare would bring. There's just something so refreshing about waking up, starting a brand new day and getting to choose how that's going to play out on a plate or in a bowl.

On a more serious note, what you eat in the morning has a ripple effect on the rest of your day. It determines the kind of energy you will experience, what moods will surface, what will be your snack foods preferences and how you metabolise the food you *do* choose for breakfast.

How is this so? Let's say you choose what a huge percentage of people reach for in the morning if they are either on the go, late for work/school run, or popping into the cafe at the station on the way to a work commute. The choice I am referring to is the 'Coffee & Muffin to go'!

Difficult to resist, is the lure of the cute little cafe blackboards sitting outside your favourite cafe, directly in your path to remind you how *important* it is to 'fuel up and get an extra muffin for free' or 'start your morning with coffee, scone and get a coffee refill for free'! But what they omit to tell you about, is the fall out from such a decision.

By giving in to the inviting promises of 'starting your day the perfect way', you have bombarded your body with the stress hormone cortisol. Cortisol itself, if over stimulated, stops the body from burning body fat. As a result, it contributes to the dreaded expanding waistline and puts the body into an aftermath of low blood sugar levels. Having low blood sugar comes with its own collection of mood swings and cravings for another shot of caffeine and sugar. And so the cycle begins. All this, as a result of the common early morning preference for so many people today.

So what would be a better option when faced with the above scenario?
If you are time poor in the morning and generally find yourself rushing out of the door with little time to catch a breath, I would firstly revisit the chapter on conscious eating. Even if you were to reach for an *organic green juice* followed by a *chia seed porridge*, as long as you are in stress mode by rushing around, no good can come of the food you eat or the drink you wash it down with. I am not suggesting that you take the weekend-style leisurely pace if you need to attend to the school run or are on your early commute schedule. Rather, it would pay in the long run to start experimenting with reshuffling your early schedule. Starting with a *sufficient* and *quality* sleep each night. If necessary, you could try waking a little earlier, allowing just enough time to give breakfast, and your digestion, the respect and honour it deserves. This way, the likelihood is that you will leave your home with a spring in your step, just like you once did in your early twenties, when life's exuberance began the moment you awoke.

If the 'Coffee and Muffin' is something you can't seem to let go of, then I am suspecting that you are fond of the *cake*-like baked food items, served with a hot beverage. My suggestion here, would be to start *gradually* including something a little healthier *alongside or* preferably *before* your current choice. For example, if you are choosing a muffin and coffee, *add in* either a piece of fresh fruit, a tablespoon of good quality nut butter, or both! *Over time*, this will set the stage for the body's desire to move towards the healthier options and will *ease out* the not so healthy ones.

There is a very valid reason for my suggesting the nut butter addition. First of all, when choosing a nut butter, it is *imperative* that you choose one without anything else added on the ingredient list, with the exception of perhaps a little sea salt.

Nut butter is my personal favourite protein fix and can transform what could potentially be a high sugar breakfast into a nutritionally balanced start to the day. It may not be as concentrated in protein content as, let's say an egg, or a piece of fish or some prime roast beef, but it's quick, nutritious, and incredibly tasty.

Speaking of fish and beef, Mum's quick and easy way to send us off to school with a satisfying glow of being 'well fed', was to get the frying pan on and either create a toast topping of three or four fish fingers or a beef burger!
I now understand why I always experienced a dull nausea on the bus journey to school. At the time I blamed it on travel sickness, coupled with a fear about not having my homework completed perfectly! I guess Mum intuitively knew that there is merit in starting the

day with protein, however, perhaps a little misguided as to what that source should be as a healthy option.

Starting the day with a good protein source will keep you satisfied for longer, without the dreaded tummy rumbles around 11am, when most people head for the cookie jar to meet a sugar fix need.

Suggested Options.
Eggs - Poached, boiled, scrambled, or baked. Yes, you *can* bake an egg!; Line a small ramekin dish with coconut oil, pop some little pieces of either veggies, anchovies or slice tomato on the bottom. Break the egg on top, cover and bake until done. Simple, quick and delicious!

Many people equate breakfast with the conventional breakfast style dishes such as cereals, yoghurt, toast, jam, coffee orange juice, etc.
There just doesn't appear to be a particular guideline out there that holds this in a *compulsory* bind. Who said we can't have veggie soup for breakfast? Chicken salad?

Why not experiment with shaking it up a little on variety, just to see what you come up with. The chances are that you will experience greater energy by swapping some traditional meals around, such as having your regular lunch time option for either breakfast or for evening meal.

If you are someone who never feels hungry enough to eat breakfast in the morning, or who really doesn't like

to eat early, you might want to reflect on how late in the evening you are eating your last meal of the day.
If you can see a pattern of eating late in the evening, or too close to bed time, that would be the first place I would recommend tweaking.

Start by having a 'closed kitchen' policy, at least two hours before bedtime. Ideally it would be better to leave three or four hours after eating before sleep, but remember, you are just starting to *tweak* here, so be patient.

It takes 21 days to change a habit! This theory has been tried and tested and makes a lot of sense.

There is something about the 'closed kitchen' approach that you may want to take note of. Having a deadline for closing the kitchen doesn't mean that you stack up your supplies to bring to the sofa, in order to munch your way through your evening's TV viewing. It means that you actually *stop eating* two, three or four hours before bedtime.

You can mark this point by brushing your teeth for example. This would be symbolic of the end of the day's intake.
If you are starting to explore this exercise, begin noticing how you feel when you wake up. Do you notice that you are beginning to feel a little hungry perhaps? or hungry earlier than you would normally? This is a good sign.

If breakfast *still* doesn't appeal to you, then gradually try easing your way into getting *something* into your digestive system , in order to start your metabolism running. This is all important if you are concerned about getting your weight into balance or to address a slowing metabolic rate due to thyroid under functioning or any other reason your metabolism might be functioning under par.

That 'something' can be as little as a crunchy green apple, a stick of celery, a slice of cucumber, or a nibble from yesterday's leftover veggie quiche (ok, that's pushing it). If however, you really want to go the extra mile, you could make yourself a nice big yummy green smoothie! After all, isn't that what everyone's doing these days??......
I'm not condemning the infamous green smoothie culture, indeed far from it. But in reality, it's not everyone's ideal start to the day, having to whip out the blender, wash a bunch of organic spinach (carefully mulling over the possibility of the occasional slug and subsequently discarding it respectfully). Then washing and chopping some celery sticks, apples and cucumber. Not forgetting also, to crack open the packet of pressed hemp seeds which were ethically sourced and legally transported through national customs and placed in your special glass jar in the refrigerator for cool storage, which will also help disguise the packet text which states 'sold as animal feed'.

Toast.

The toast itself, *providing there are no sensitivities to gluten*, is best made from bread sourced fresh from a local bakery. If you suspect that you might have some gluten sensitivities, try a good sourdough bread, as the fermentation processing is less detrimental to the gut than regular bread.   Bakery fresh bread will most often be void of the extensive list of preservatives and additives, sugars and additional questionable ingredients that make up many of the factory baked varieties.

What about those who are celiac or have severe sensitivities to gluten?
The gluten free options can be a tricky one to get right. It's not that there is a shortage of gluten free options out there. In fact gluten free products are springing up in abundance everywhere.
Upon close inspection of the ingredient list on many gluten free options, you may unfortunately find that they contain copious ingredients of questionable necessity, with the majority of which, if eaten to excess, can be downright detrimental to your health.

Simple is best and less is more. Isn't that what our mothers for generations have been telling us? (unless of course you are referring to my Mum's home baked creamy rice pudding...*Chapter 5*).

My personal toppings of choice.
Nut Butter; - any of the following; Peanut (containing just peanuts! nothing else, sea salt at most) / Almond / Almond & Peanut / Almond, Brazil & Cashew / Cashew.

Nut butters are a great way to sneak in a healthy protein if you are a vegetarian or if you just want to simplify breakfast preparation.

On top of that I like to spread a *little **pure honey*** (I like raw un pasteurised honey as it has not gone through a heating process and therefore retains its amazing immunity boosting health properties).
The reason I spread just a *little,* is because of the sugar issue which I touched on earlier. But isn't good honey healthy? Yes it is, but when it goes into the body, along with all the goodness, the body processes it as sugar. Again, less is more.
By using just adequate to receive the benefit, and by adding a protein such as nut butter which helps to avoid the blood sugar spike, the result is delicious and nutritious.
The additional topping options I choose are, a ***sprinkling of cinnamon*** and a generous helping of ***frozen berries*** (taken out of the freezer the night before so they are soft and succulent).

If I am in a more 'savoury' mood, I will spread some ***real butter*** or ***avocado.*** I may even top this too with some berries! I never wandered far from the sweet and savoury combinations.

I believe it may have stemmed from home cooked Christmas Dinner, and the yearly appearance of Cranberry Sauce. The jar would appear on Christmas Day and would remain on the table at all mealtimes until February or March! Cranberry sauce with everything from eggs, to beans on toast!

Back to breakfast.

Some of the more traditional toppings, which I like to save for the weekends when void of clock watching, are as follows:

Eggs! As I mentioned earlier, eggs are a convenient and super healthy protein.

Many people mistakenly discard the yolks. That's is equivalent to buying a new pair of shoes and throwing away the sole!

The egg is perfectly formed, providing of course that the bird it came from was not caged and/or fed hormones, or genetically modified corn feed. Plus that it had a happy life roaming around as life intended. So if you are having an egg, have the egg, all of it! High in protein, essential omega 3 fats, Vitamin E, A & K, and the necessary brain for functioning-cholesterol. Eggs will leave you feeling totally satisfied for the rest of the morning until lunchtime, avoiding the need for high sugar and/or caffeine quick fixes.

Lunch.

Lunch largely depends on what your situation is and where you are when lunch comes around.

A little word of warning though, if you are either working from home, a stay-home Mum or on a home-during-the-day schedule, give yourself a deadline as to when lunch starts and when lunch finishes.

From personal experience, this strategy must be mastered as quickly as possible, to avoid the extended lunchtime continuous grazing that can leave you bloated, tired, grumpy and unenthusiastic about completing remaining tasks.

I recommend scheduling something to do, preferably something active, as soon as lunch is finished(taking note of the aforementioned lunch cut off time). Failing to do this will leave you open to procrastination, apathy, boredom, and/or emotional eating.
If you are an emotional eater, then refer back to 'conscious eating' chapter and re-run through the guidelines to address this.

When deciding what to have for lunch, apart from taking into consideration your situation and location at lunchtime, it's a good idea to think about what your upcoming afternoon schedule is like.
This refers to the relationship between *what* you eat and *how you feel afterwards*.
My earlier reference to the typical blow-out Sunday lunch or Christmas fare, or Thanksgiving spread, shows evidence of this equation and the subsequent desire to sleep.
So have a look at what the afternoon is likely to consist of by way of tasks, activities and/or errands to run, and gage the lunch content accordingly.

Originally a British tradition, **Baked Beans** which are regularly served on toast and often a lunchtime favourite, have remained a favourite for me too. I have however, created my own relatively healthier version which is now a family favourite.

My recipe has evolved substantially from opening a can of already manufactured beans in tomato sauce and heating in a saucepan, to the following;

Ingredients & Method.

Onion(chopped)
Olive oil(providing it is not heated to a very high temperature, alternatively use avocado oil or coconut oil)
Sea salt & black pepper(sprinkled before serving).
Tomato Puree
Beans such as *cannellini, black, brown, pinto or navy* (strained and rinsed through sieve)

Stir fry onion until soft.
Add jar of tomato puree (preferably one that contains just tomato, with no sugar added).
Allow sauce to reduce until relatively thick. Add strained and rinsed beans.
Stir well until heated, then serve.

Suggestions for serving:
With **grated cheese** on top / On **Toast** (traditional)/ As a topping for baked **kumara**(sweet potato) / With **rice** or **mashed potatoes**.

As an advocate for the convenience, nutritional value and delicious taste of legumes (peas, beans, lentils), I reach for these little miraculous wonders on a regular basis. They have become a staple in our home for many quick and easy twenty minute 'pot to plate' dishes.

Here are some of the additional ways I use them in my one pan wonders.

Stewp.
I couldn't quite decide whether to create a soup or a stew so I decided to just start with the basics and let it evolve authentically. The result evolved as a deliciously filling and nutritionally abundant *stewp*.

Foundation ingredients.

*Onions, garlic, herbs & spices (*combination of cumin, coriander, turmeric, a little chilli(fresh or dried).
For a more mediterranean style flavour, use a combination of oregano, basil, rosemary, sage & thyme. My choice of vegetables for these dishes will vary depending on what I have in the fridge at the time. *Anything goes!*

Some may prefer to separate some vegetable options, but through experimentation, the more variety of vegetables you are getting your kids and family to consume daily, you are heading down the healthy road and that, in itself, makes my heart sing.

On the topic of vegetables, I would recommend staying as much as possible within the varieties that are *in season* and *grown locally.* Adhering to this theory provides enhanced flavour and supports local farmers as a result. Naturally, in winter months, nature does provide the more dense varieties, which are nurturing, grounding, warming and filling.

Then when the warmer months roll around, nature provides the lighter varieties, such as spring greens, leafy greens, celery, capsicum and courgettes.
Both dense and lighter vegetables combine really well with the assortment of beans/legumes I have recommended above.

As it is a *one pan* dish, add your choice of vegetables once the onions, garlic and spices/herbs have been sautéed for a few minutes.
Then add the beans, peas/legumes for the remaining cooking time.

The overall cooking time will vary according to the vegetables chosen. This is one you just need to keep an eye on and judge according to your texture preference.
For **meat** eaters, one pan dishes are also a quick and easy option.
Replace the legumes with your choice of cubed/diced **beef**, **chicken** or **lamb** etc.
As the meat will take a little longer to cook, I would add this prior to the vegetables and quite soon after the onions and garlic.

If you like to create a **sauce** consistency to the above suggestions, here are my two most often created.
Tomato : using jar of tomato puree, added to vegetables and reduced until the required consistency.
Peanut sauce : I would prefer to make this in a separate pot and then either add to the mix or serve drizzled on top.
Heat approximately 1 cup of milk (either cows milk, almond milk, rice milk, or soy milk) in a small pan. Add

a splash of tomato ketchup, (even the healthiest of pantries will have a bottle of ketchup in its midst!), a splash of tamari soy sauce and a good tablespoon of peanut butter.

Stir until reduced into a sauce consistency and either add to the mix or drizzle on top.

The above suggestions, can be served either by itself, or on a bed of additional greens. Alternatively for a heartier accompaniment, it may be served with Rice, Pasta, Bulgar Wheat or Cous Cous. Gluten free options are Quinoa, Millet, Buckwheat, Rice Pasta or Rice Noodles.

One more versatile and easy to put together dishes is my *salad combos.*

I have a newfound respect for the magical power of the Food Processor.

I was reluctant to succumb to the trend of the Food Processing kitchen assistant, as I believed that the preparation of food is that of a meditative exercise and therefore should be carried out in a slow and methodical manner.

I eventually realised that it was in no way disrespectful of the food, if I were to have a mechanical assistant for preparation. Instead, it was in fact letting go an element of undercurrent 'time stress'.

So with the food processor at the ready, here are some combinations that I love to create in my time saving salad bowls.

Remember, any of these can be mixed and matched according to your personal preference and food at hand.

In the following combinations, I just place the washed vegetables into the processor and switch on for as long as it takes to create the consistency I require. A shorter time is required if you like bigger chunks and likewise, longer if you like them in a breadcrumb like texture.

*** Carrot / Red & or Yellow Beet / Apple / Celery**

*** Carrot / Celery / Fennel / Apple**

*** Carrot / Red Beet / Red onion / Red Capsicum(Bell Pepper)**

*** White Cabbage / Carrot / Spring onion / Radish**

*** White Cabbage / Red Cabbage / Fennel / Green Capsicum / Fresh chilli (tiny piece)**

Any and all of the above can have a sprinkling of seeds and/or nuts, such as; *Chia / Sunflower / Pumpkin / Crushed Walnuts / Shaved Almonds / Grated Brazil Nut*

Any and all of the above can have a little sweetness added by sprinkling a few *raisins* through, once processed.

Dressings can either be added through the mix or individually upon serving.

Dressing options.

* Olive oil & sea salt

* Olive Oil & Balsamic Vinegar, Sea Salt & crushed Black Pepper

** Toasted Sesame oil & Brown Rice Vinegar
Olive oil, Wholegrain Mustard, Honey, White Rice Vinegar, Sea salt & crushed Black Pepper*

* Umoboshi Vinegar & Avocado Oil (use Umoboshi vinegar sparingly as it tastes quite salty).

Having just scratched the surface as far as recipes go, I do hope that I have perhaps opened the door for you to step through and create your own masterpieces, using the basics.

Cooking is something that needs to be embraced authentically, with respect and with a lot of love. It doesn't have to be flash, clever, a work of art, or a dish to top all others. It just needs to come from the heart, knowing that what is going on the plates of you and your family, will be an energy that goes beyond the replenishing of your cells and the strengthening of your bones.

My Italian friend, a chef, who cooked in my favourite cafe in the North of England, put it so beautifully when I once asked him;

"Stef, what's in this soup, it's just superb?" His response was....

*"A little bit tomato....A little bit vegetable...A little bit herbs ...An' A **Lotta Love**"!*

12. What does Happy look like?

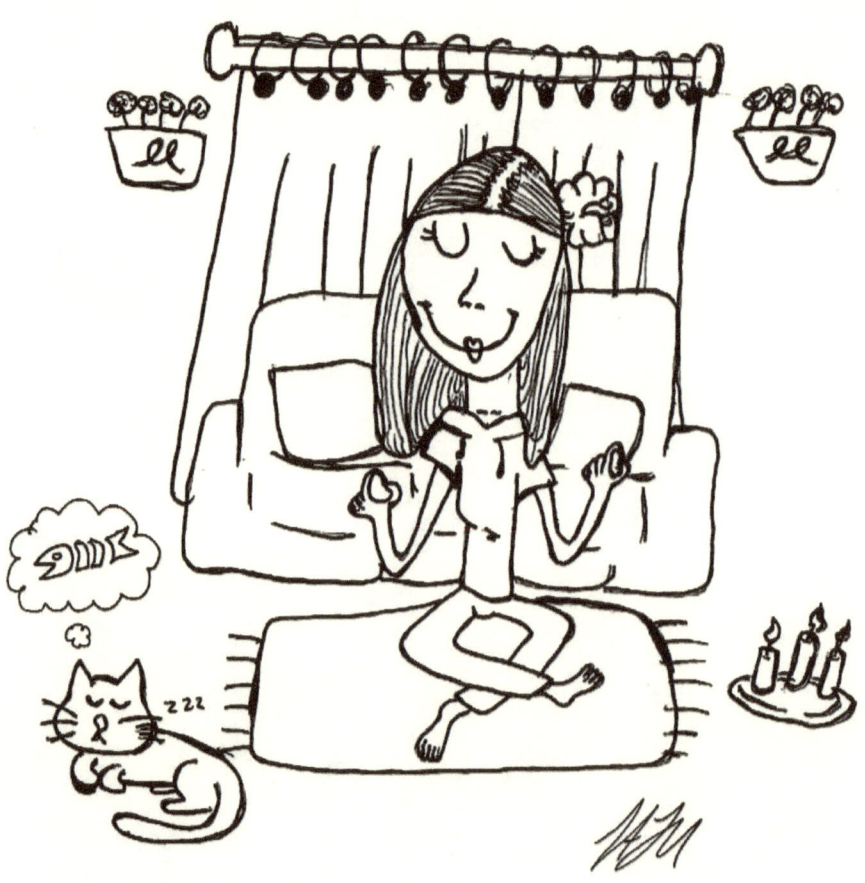

As I began writing this chapter, I was experiencing a clash of emotions. The most predominant emotion was that of happiness. I had just experienced the pure joy of listening to my daughter's sweet renditions of her day at school. She was excitedly over loaded with the urgency of her little dramas. I smiled as I listened, and I knew in that moment I was experiencing happiness in all its simplicity.

When that moment was over, I returned to the complex and interwoven blends of frustration and irritation. Frustration because of the sudden disappearance of the few paragraphs I had already crafted for this chapter and the irritation that my computer was still playing hide and seek with my work.

It is so easy to shift from happiness to something that is conflicting with happiness, but that isn't necessarily a negative experience. It is the authentic unfolding of a regular day, in the life of a regular human existence.

It is often mistakenly believed, that happiness is to be experienced consistently and in order to achieve this there must be something which, once engaged in, flicks the inner switch and turns on your 'happy heart'.

I can confidently speculate, that when asked what it would take to create happiness in the average person's life, this would be met with an array of conditions. Conditions such as;
more money, a better job, a bigger house, a successful career, a better partner, a car, a yacht. The list is potentially endless.

Looking at these conditions, if probed with the question "what do you want by getting what you want"?, ultimately the answer would almost always be "to be happy".

As is well documented in the media, with evidence showing up from the celebrity world, having all of that, and more, does not necessarily make you happy.

We have all no doubt, been on our own personal quest to find that ultimate happy place. Each one, setting out on the same quest and choosing our individual route to get there. Scrambling, fumbling, stumbling and occasionally finding a glimmer, if only for a fleeting moment.

I recall my own personal quest for that eluded state of permanent euphoria. I am reminded of the sentiment that my dear Mum would end each telephone conversation with. I dialled in from all corners of the globe, providing her with a low down on my latest adventure, upcoming course, recent certification or enthusiasm about my latest entrepreneurial ideas. Mum listened on in what I can only guess was complete confusion and/or oblivion, to the importance or understanding of what any of it was all about. Once I had offloaded my musings, she closed the conversation on each occasion with "Ah well, as long as you're happy"...
Back then, I didn't put much emphasis on this sentiment, but now I can clearly see how these words came, not only to guide me, but to let me know that I didn't have to

be or do anything, or change who I was in order to be happy. I just needed to decide that whatever situation I chose to be in, I can also make that choice to be happy no matter what.

There are certain cliches that create a little confusion around what it takes to be really happy, especially when relating to money and happiness. *"Money can't buy you happiness" "If only I had……..then I'd be happy"* and *"You can't be happy all the time!"*.

Whilst money certainly does not buy happiness, it can definitely help you create an environment that can afford you security, peace of mind and freedom. So whilst it cannot buy you happiness itself, it can, *if used productively*, be a catalyst for laying the foundation to creating that happy and secure place within.

How often have you waited for something to happen, for something to change or for something to be added to your collection of items, only to find that the anticipated euphoria was for the most part flat and anticlimactic? I have been in this situation countless times, anticipating the 'what ifs' and the 'if only' scenarios.

Today, I am less inclined to rely upon someone other than myself, to arrange my circumstances in a bid for resulting happiness.

Taking this kind of responsibility is not a practice which comes easily. In fact, it does require digging deep and opening up to a mindset of consciousness.

So what does happy look like for *you?* What is *your own* version of happy?

Explore it, reflect on it, then go out there and *create it*. Be the one who makes you smile and be the one who supports you through your darkest moments.

So much in present day has been written on the subject of happiness, much of which has been depicted from the early sages, philosophers and wise words of some of the world's most respected leaders.
So I am not about to re-invent the wheel by delving into the programming and re-programming of your subconscious minds. I am however, going to present you with 50 pocket sized and *doable* little guidelines, which you can choose to implement *over time,* in which order you prefer.

I hope that as you make your way through the list, you will recognise some of what you are incorporating in your life already. I hope that some guidelines will also inspire you to begin them today, and if inclined, share with those whose lives you wish to add a sparkle of joy to and to the lives of their loved ones.

These are guidelines which I have personally adopted at one point or another throughout my journey so far. They have impacted me on some level in a positive way, and I hope they will do the same for you.

1. Be grateful, for everything, especially the little things that are easily taken for granted (such as the ability to hold this book in your hands and read it).

2. Wear the best quality underwear you can afford.

3. Listen attentively to the little stories your child(ren) tell you.

4. Ask for help.

5. Always keep your footwear in good condition.

6. Be polite and kind to your neighbours, you just never know when you may need their help.

7. Light a candle when having dinner, even if, and especially when, you are dining alone.

8. Smile when you answer the phone, the energy travels more than you think.

9. Offer at least one compliment per day.

10. When you feel the world is against you, seek out someone who needs your help and do what you can for them.

11. When choosing chocolate, go for the best quality you can find.

12. Drink water when struggling to make a decision.

13. Leave little endearing notes or smilies on the bathroom mirror for your loved one(s) to find.

14. Always hug your child(ren) before they leave the house to go to school.

15. Switch technology off during all mealtimes.

16. Always listen, undistracted by technology, to anyone whom you are having a conversation with.

17. Support local businesses as much as possible.

18. Give to charity, no matter how little, even if, and especially if, you think you can't afford it.

19. Keep your car neat, tidy & clean, inside and out (your car is an extension of how you represent yourself).

20. De clutter at every opportunity (this saves time on a 'big clean sweep').

21. Sign a 'thank you' note on every bill as you pay it before filing it away.

22. Compliment and acknowledge yourself for your greatness, daily.

23. Mail little impromptu cards with thoughtful wishes, either bought or self-made, to those who have touched your life in a positive way (via snail mail which requires a postage stamp!).

24. Switch off your mobile phone on every car journey, no matter how short the distance.

25. Leave your bedroom in the morning in exactly the state you would like to see it in the evening.

26. Open all windows in the morning, regardless of the season.

27. Be polite to waiters, shop assistants and anyone in the service industry whom you come in contact with.

28. Spend quiet time in the morning, no matter how rushed you think you are, to breathe, contemplate and give gratitude.

29. Move, stretch and bend your body daily.

30. Eat a variety of foods from all food groups.

31. Forgive everyone, including and especially, yourself.

32. Allow the sun to grace your bare skin, in summer and in winter.

33. Sing often, even if you think you can't hold a note.

34. Dance often, even if you think you have two left feet.

35. If you *feel* something isn't right, it probably isn't (your intuition is guiding you).

34. Say 'no' to what does not inspire you.

35. Say 'yes' to what you really want.

36. Choose what's right instead of what's popular.

37. Give a homeless person a food item instead of money.

38. Clean the corners of your home regularly.

39. Wake up early every day, even on days off and holidays.

40. Ensure your bedroom is in complete darkness when sleeping.

41. Learn, learn, and keep learning, forever.

42. Eat something raw with every meal.

43. Welcome new neighbours with a small gift or with something you have baked.

44. Have a smile ready for everyone you meet, whether you know them or not.

45. Learn to love sauerkraut.

46. Be punctual, always.

47. Be courteous to everyone, especially the elderly.

48. Accept feedback graciously and with thanks.

49. Love Your Mum.

50. Love your Dad.

As I close this chapter, I will leave you with the words of Marci Shimoff, author of *'Happy for no Reason'*.....

"May you be safe, may you be happy, may you be healthy and may you live with ease"....

. . . .

www.ingramcontent.com/pod-product-compliance
Lightning Source LLC
Chambersburg PA
CBHW020531290526
45786CB00002B/831